Identification of Drugs
in
Pharmaceutical Formulations
by
Thin Layer Chromatography

SECOND EDITION

Identification of Drugs
in
Pharmaceutical Formulations
by
Thin Layer Chromatography

SECOND EDITION

Editor

Dr. P.D. SETHI

M.Pharm., Ph.D.

Pharmaceutical Analyst, New Delhi, India

Associate Editor

Dilip CHAREGAONKAR

M.Sc.

Anchrom HPTLC Application Laboratory,
Mumbai, India

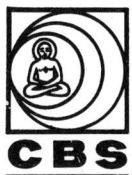

CBS

CBS PUBLISHERS & DISTRIBUTORS PVT. LTD.

New Delhi • Bengaluru • Chennai • Kochi • Mumbai • Pune

ISBN : 81-239-0635-8

First Edition : 1992
Second Edition : 1999
Reprint : 2003, 2004, 2005, 2008, 2010, 2014

Published by Satish Kumar Jain and produced by V.K. Jain for CBS Publishers & Distributors Pvt. Ltd.,
CBS Plaza, 4819/XI Prahlad Street, 24 Ansari Road, Daryaganj, New Delhi - 110002, India.   • Website: www.cbspd.com
e-mail: delhi@cbspd.com, cbspubs@airtelmail.in
Ph.: 23289259, 23266861, 23266867   • Fax: 011-23243014

Branches:

• *Bengaluru:* Seema House, 2975, 17th Cross, K.R. Road,
  Bansankari 2nd Stage, Bengaluru - 560070
    • Ph.: +91-80-26771678/79 • Fax: +91-80-26771680
    • E-mail: cbsbng@gmail.com, bangalore@cbspd.com
• *Pune:* Bhuruk Prestige, Sr. No. 52/12/2+1+3/2,
  Narhe, Haveli (Near Katraj-Dehu Road By-pass), Pune - 411041
    • Ph.: +91-20-64704058/59   • E-mail: pune@cbspd.com
• *Kochi:* 36/14, Kalluvilakam, Lissie Hospital Road,
  Kochi - 682018, Kerala • Ph.: +91-484-4059061-65
    • Fax: +91-484-4059065   • E-mail: cochin@cbspd.com
• *Chennai:* 20, West Park Road, Shenoy Nagar, Chennai - 600030
  Ph.: +91-44-26260666, 26208620   • Fax: +91-44-42032115
    • E-mail: chennai@cbspd.com
• *Mumbai:* 83-C, Dr. E. Moses Road, Worli, Mumbai-400 018, Maharashtra
  Ph.: +91-9833017933   • E-mail: mumbai@cbspd.com

Printed at :
J.S. Offset Printers, Delhi

Thin-Layer Chromatography

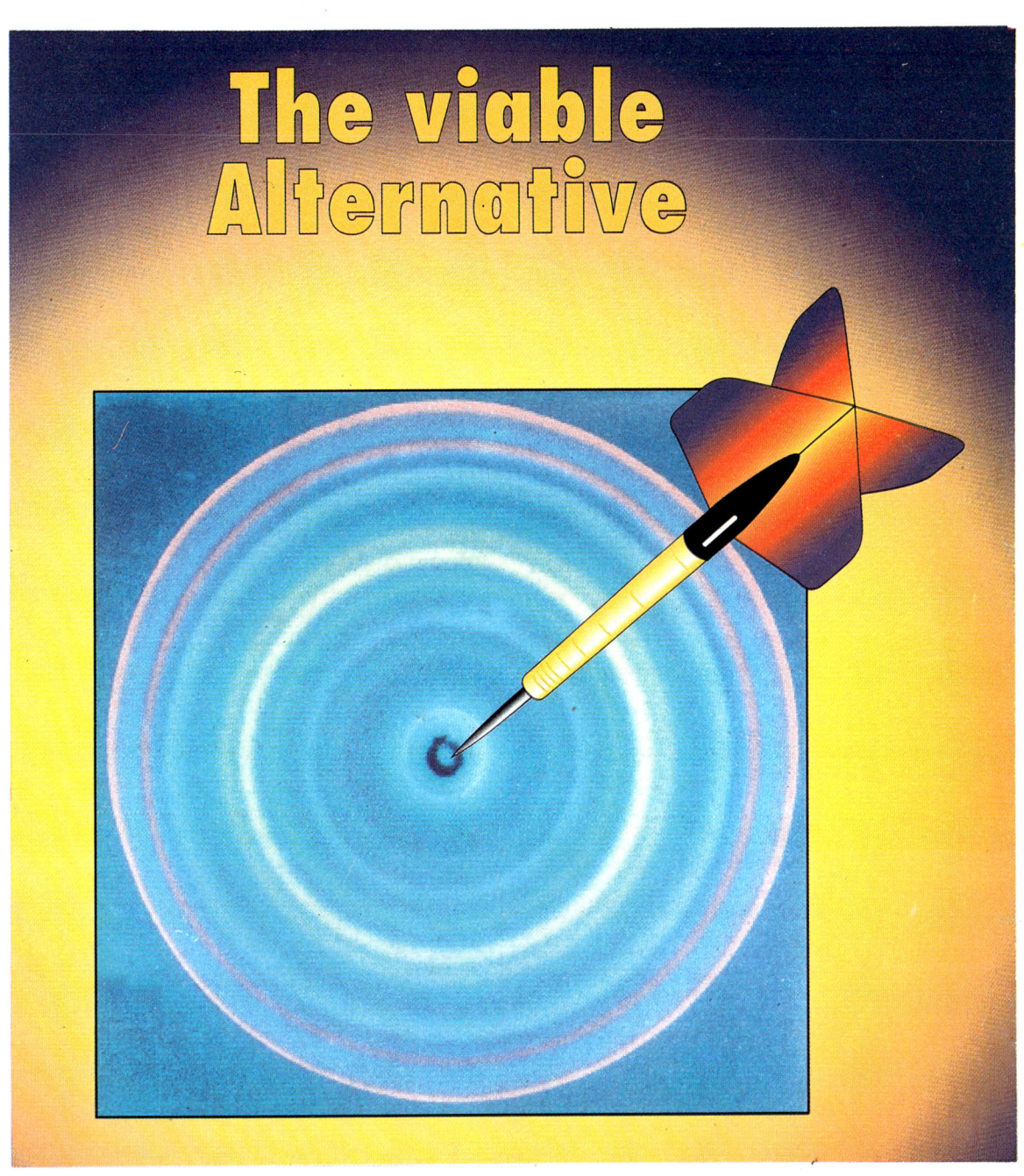

The viable Alternative

Dedicated to Fellow Analysts

"No serious effort in life is totally accomplished by oneself, this book is no exception."

Preface to the Second Edition

All the official compendias now include detailed monograph on Thin Layer Chromatography technique primarily for purpose of identification and for assessing low level of impurities/related substances or decomposition products in a drug substance.

Most important use of Thin Layer Chromatography is to identify the unknown sample components or to confirm the identity of the analyte. It can serve as a screening step followed by HPLC confirmation and quantitation of only positive samples which results in lower analytical time and cost compared with analysis of all samples by HPLC.

To have highest confidence in the identification procedure, R_f values of the spot/zone from the sample should be compared with standard analyte in more than one type of TLC system with different separation mechanism such as normal and reversed phase. Alternatively, multiple solvent system may be used with one type of layer.

The revised text describes the procedures for separation and identification of each component in 172 divergent multi-component formulations using both normal and RP sorbent layers. To enhance the usefulness of this technique, most of the formulations contain several alternate mobile phases and sorbent layers for analysts to choose from and optimise.

Qualitative identification is primarily based on characteristic colour produced by a specific reagent combined with R_f values. Identification may be further aided by the use of more than one detection reagent. With post-chromatographic derivatization as tool for detection and identification, TLC is a versatile technique. This is normally achieved by spraying or dipping the developed chromatogram into solution of the reagent, followed by air drying or heating.

The revised edition includes a comprehensive chapter on detection/visualization reagents most commonly used for post-chromatographic derivatization of substances of pharmaceutical interest. Detailed composition and method for preparation of each reagent has been described. The reagent may cause spots/zones to absorb visible or UV radiations or to become fluorescent for organic molecules in general or to react selectively with particular class of compounds such as diazotization reaction for aromatic amines. Gibb's reagent for phenolic substances, ninhydrin giving different colours with amino acids, iodine and sulphuric acid being the universal reagents are often employed in the text. Each reagent has been listed with drugs which can possibly be detected with the reagent.

The authors would like to express their appreciation of analysts who continue to be source of inspiration. The authors express their gratitude towards Mr. Satish Kumar Jain and Mr. Vinod Kumar Jain for their continuous support in publication of the revised edition. We are ever grateful to Shri Dharmvir for his excellent execution of the project.

The author (Dr. P.D. Sethi) is indebted to his wife Usha for checking and comparing the manuscript, and for her moral support and inspiration without which my various contributions in the field of "Pharmaceutical Analysis" would never have been possible.

P.D. SETHI
DILIP CHAREGAONKAR

Preface to the First Edition

The majority of the methods originate from the needs of certain field of science. Thin Layer Chromatography (TLC) was first used by Ismailov and Shraiber for the analysis of alkaloids in plant extracts. Its rediscovery by E. Stahl arose from the need of pharmaceutical laboratories. In view of the application of this technique in various branches of science, we cannot but see the increasingly growing number of pharmaceutical applications. While considering the question of standardising this technique from the beginning of its history, the work done by E. Stahl is to be deeply appreciated.

Identification is pre-requisite before proceeding with quantitation. Identification of each component in commercially available multi-component formulations is extremely difficult as, most of the time, pharmacopoeial identification tests are not answered in such combinations due to mutual interference. When other methods of identification fail, TLC may serve the purpose on account of its extreme selectivity and rapidity. I like the TLC much more than LC and HPLC, because I can see chromatogram, the important feature of TLC, the visual experience (almost 90% of all the information we gather reaches us through our visual sense). The characterisation of the spot such as its colour and shape or colour with different spray reagents at various temperatures are usually unique for a compound. All these observations add to the experimental data and enhance our confidence in our results.

Thin layer chromatography is one of the indispensable techniques available which can be used as an independent method or in combination with other methods complementing and enhancing one another. To summarize everything about application of TLC would be an unachievable goal and beyond the scope of this book. I have devoted my attention to the type of drug formulations which are commonly being marketed at present. The Rf values multiplied by hundred, so called hRf values, are only approximate, indicating the relative mobility of the compounds in the chromatogram. Other experimental conditions like chamber saturation state, length of run, separation technique, adsorbent used and preparation of plates have been maintained uniformly throughout. The procedure for preparation of the sample and quantity to be applied is described for each formulation in individual chromatogram. For occasional thin layer chromatographic work, a side laboratory fitted with a table or bench to support the developing tank and a fume cupboard for detection is quite adequate, in such cases pre-coated plates may be used.

In a busy chromatographic testing laboratory, it is advantageous to set up a full-fledged chromatographic unit. Design with complete layout for occasional TLC work as well as for a well planned TLC laboratory has been described. However, the design must of course be harmonised with the aim of the work and characteristics of the place. The most salient features of the text is that it includes two different solvent systems, so called universal solvent systems I and II which have been applied for the identification of different components in as many as 82 and 28 drug formulations of different categories respectively. The chromatograms have been arranged in order of therapeutic use of the formulations such as analgesics and antipyretics, anthelmintics, anti-allergics, antibiotics, anti-diarrhoeals, anti-emetics, anti-inflammatory, anti-malarials, anti-spasmodics, anti-tuberculous, bronchospasm relaxants, expectorants, keratolytics and cleansers, sedatives and tranquillisers, urinary anti-infective and miscellaneous. The text describes chromatographic behaviour of 126 drug substances.

My main aim is to demonstrate how TLC fits in a well managed analytical laboratory as an indispensable technique on its own. When I joined this laboratory, my experience about TLC was mere surface veneer and consequently I learnt a great deal and this book distils what I have learnt at the bench during last one decade. I had this unique opportunity to learn from my fellow analysts how to blend objective facts and subjective intuition into something that could perhaps be termed the process of thinking. The analytical data may be dealt with by computers or human intellect, the intuition is exclusively human. Whenever, these two factors merge in right proportion, we have the most powerful combination for advancement of science. The information contained in this book is to create a framework for experimentation necessary to generate identification profile for drug formulations. Since most of the work presented in this text is based on actual laboratory experiments, the data is most unpublished.

It may be interesting to add that most of the systems described in the text are routinely being used in the laboratory with excellent results for identification of compounds as a substitute for compendial tests. The methods and results presented in this book may not be the only one available and better alternatives may well exist, however, it should provide a worthwhile beginning and it is left to the future authors to improve upon my endeavours. After all, it is the countless anomalies which make our endeavour so interesting.

"A man would do nothing if he waited until he could do it so well, that no one would find fault with what he had done."

The author is grateful to Dr. Y.K.S. Rathor, Dr. S.C. Mathur and Dr. N. Murgesan for their excellent assistance in preparation of manuscript. The author wishes to express his most sincere gratitude to Dr. O.P. Ghai for his continuous guidance. The author shall always remain indebted to his wife Usha for moral support throughout his career.

P.D. SETHI

Contents

SETTING UP YOUR TLC LAB

- Silica gel precoated TLC plates in aluminium, glass and plastic
- TLC modified (RP-8, RP-18, NH_2, CN, Diol, Chiral) and impregnated layers
- Microcapillaries / syringes for spotting sample
- Development chambers
- Iodine chamber
- TLC glass sprayer
- Ready to use spraying solutions
- UV lamp 254 nm and 366 nm
- Reference substances
- Literature on application

Thin Layer Chromatography

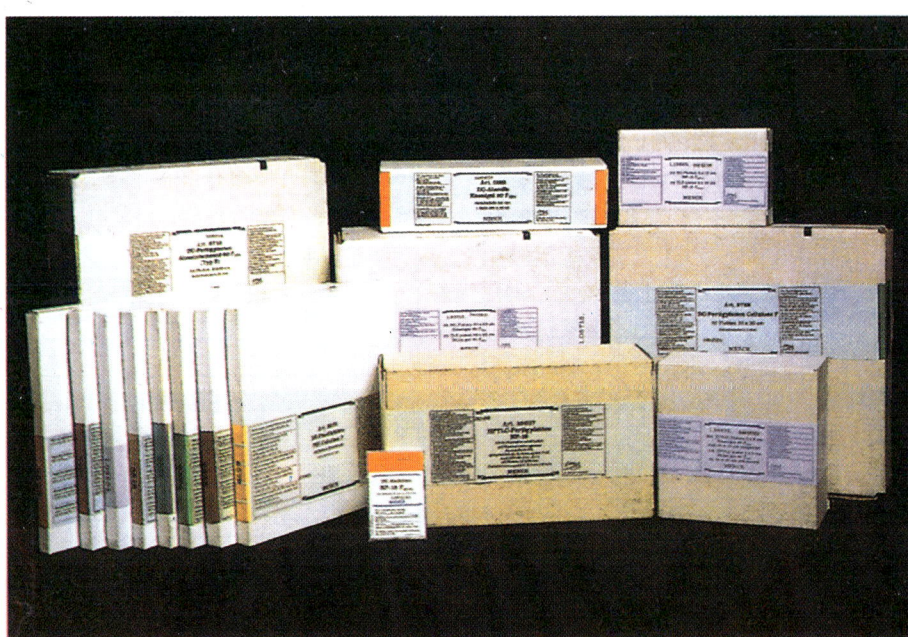

- Si
- RP-2
- RP-8
- RP-18
- NH_2
- CN
- DIOL
- Al Oxide
- Cellulose
- Chiral

Specialities :

- GLP coded
- Concentration zone
- Multiformat plates
- With acid resistant fluorescent indicator

Wide range of pre-coated Plates to suit your needs

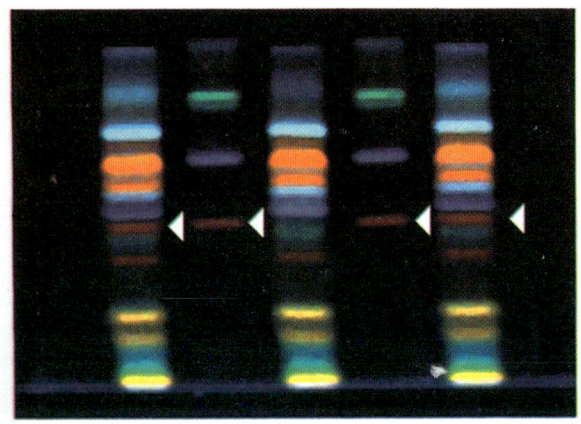

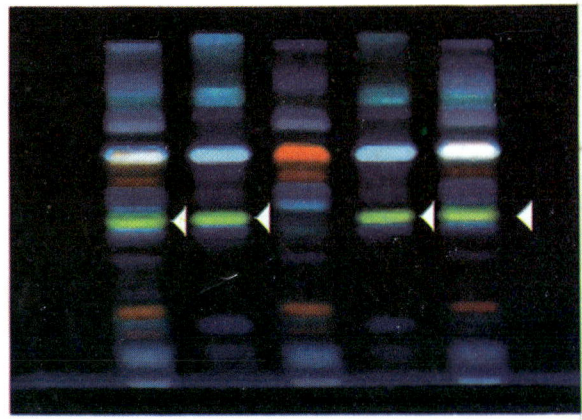

Introduction

Identification is prerequisite before proceeding with quantitation. Thin layer chromatography is one of the most widely used techniques for rapid identification of drugs and its formulations. It is equality applicable to drugs in their pure state, to those extracted from pharmaceutical formulations and to biological samples. There are several reasons for the practical use of this technique :

- Simple to learn and perform, always available for use since precoated plates are usually employed without any further preparation.
- The time required to demonstrate the presence of constituents of drug formulations by TLC is very short.
- The method is economical as the solvent consumption is small and there is virtually no waste disposal problem. The method of detection does not place any restriction on the choice of mobile phase.
- In addition to qualitative detection, TLC also provides visual semi-quantitative information on the chief active constituents of drug or drug preparations, thus enabling quick assessment of its quality.
- Wide range of possible layers in conjunction with different solvent systems allows infinite separating power.
- TLC provides a chromatographic drug finger-print, it is, therefore, suitable for monitoring the identity and purity of drugs and to detect adulteration and substitution.
- It allows possibility of separating wide classes of drugs and is surprisingly versatile in its various fields of application.
- TLC chromatogram can be documented and kept permanently in the record.
- With the aid of an appropriate separation procedure and instrumentation, TLC can be used to quantify drug combinations.

It continues to retain favour with the analysts because it is simple, reliable and economical and offers selectivity of detection through various location procedures. The technique is so flexible in the choice of stationary and mobile phases that it can be adapted to meet the requirement of each task. However, it has lower sensitivity and resolution than other popular chromatographic techniques such as GC, HPLC, but with the advent of HPTLC, these disadvantages have been reduced to a great extent.

The most valuable use of thin layer chromatography in pharmaceutical work is to provide means of assessing low levels of impurities in medicinal substances. For this purpose, the substance is applied to the chromatographic surface and, after chromatography, any secondary spots to be seen in the chromatogram after appropriate visualization are compared to size and intensity with those of low loadings of expected impurities that have simultaneously been subjected to chromatography on the same plate. Such a procedure requires that the expected impurities be available and in certain monographs the use of authentic specimens of impurities is called for. Frequently, such impurities are not available and in such cases it is often possible to compare secondary spots arising from trace impurities with the spot obtained by carrying out chromatography on the same plate using an appropriately low loading of the substance being examined. This expedient is not always possible since impurities and the substance being examined may respond in different ways to the method of detection used, but it often provides an acceptable criterion by which the level of impurity in the substance may be judged. A third procedure that is sometimes advocated is to apply such an amount of the substance being examined that, after chromatography, no secondary spots will appear if the sample is acceptably pure. This is the least satisfactory of the three methods since ability to see a secondary spot is a subjective matter and because the intensity of spots on a chromatogram may vary considerably from one occasion to another depending on the exact conditions of chromatography.

As an adjunct to identification, thin layer chromatography may be used by comparing the behaviour of the material to be identified with that of a standard substance, usually an authentic specimen of the substance being examined. If the two substances move identical distances during chromatographic process and if the two substances, when mixed together and then subjected to chromatography, move as a single substance, it may be presumed that the two substances are identical. This presumption may be strengthened by repeating the procedure using a different system of chromatography; in general, if two substances behave identically in as many as three fundamentally different systems the presumption of identity becomes very strong.

Although, the use of reference substances improve the reproducibility of the TLC system, the other chromatographic conditions should also be standardised to increase the reproducibility further. Apart from the obvious need to use pure solvents and mixtures made accurately, they should be changed once in a day if they contain solvent of different volatilities or if they are hygroscopic. The plate should be of good quality and stored in condition of constant humidity. Whatever the nature of the solvents used to apply the test substance to the plate, it must be removed by drying in a stream of warm air before the plate is transferred to the tank for development. This is especially necessary if the extract is used that may contain water. Tanks should always have paper lining and sufficient time should be allowed to enable solvents of different polarities reach equilibrium. If the substances analysed have sufficient different Rf values, the above factor may not interfere in separation, but in case of substances having close and similar mobility, these can significantly influence separation.

As nearly all the drugs of interest cannot be detected in visible radiation, they are located by means of their response to ultraviolet light and their reaction with various spray reagents. Majority of the substances can be detected by general reactions such as carbonization with sulphuric acid, exposure to iodine vapours, detection of radioactivity in case of labelled compounds or microbiological response to antibiotics.

TLC/HPTLC possess following advantages over column chromatography :

- The substances that remain at the start during chromatography under chosen conditions can easily be recognised.

- Decomposition of analyte during chromatographic development can be detected by two-dimensional TLC.

- Use of corrosive and UV absorbing mobile phases is feasible as detection is preceded by complete removal of mobile phase by evaporation.
- Substances can be detected/identified by using universal detection/visualization reagents (iodine vapours, methanolic sulphuric acid) or selective reagents.
- High sample throughput as similar or different nature of samples can be simultaneously analysed on a single plate.
- No time and material consuming regeneration steps are required as disposable TLC plates are commercially available.
- Sample clean up is often either unnecessary or necessary to a very limited degree.
- Co-TLC is possible.
- Analyst can prepare the plates in the laboratory by using loose powdered sorbent material easily available commercially.
- No carry over, hence no contamination.
- No memory effect.
- Multiple development and scanning after each development possible.
- Quality of separation can be continuously monitored as whole chromatogram can be seen at a glance.
- Formation of artifacts is rare.
- Different development techniques (vertical, horizontal, multiple, two-dimensional, continuous, circular, anticircular) possible.

Criteria for identification of an analyte by TLC

1. Rf value of an analyte should agree within ±3% compared to standard material used under similar conditions.
2. Visual appearance of the analyte should be indistinguishable from that of standard material.
3. Centre of the spot nearest to that due to analyte should be separated from it by at least half the sum of analyte spot diameter.
4. For confirming the identity, co-chromatography is mandatory. As a result, only the spot supposed to be due to analyte should be visible and no additional spot should appear.
5. Whenever spectrum detection is used, maximum absorption wavelength of the sample and standard should be same within limits of resolution of detection system and UV spectra should not be visibly different from that of the standard material.

What thin layer chromatography can accomplish?

TLC compares well with other chromatographic methods, details can be found in literature. In the present introductory text, it is important to know in what cases thin layer chromatography is particularly well suited, in contrast to other methods. If you answer one or more of the following questions in the affirmative, then you should be using TLC.

1. Do you want to see the entire chromatographic separation at a glance, with an opportunity to judge the quality of the separation, estimate the rough proportions of substances present, and recognize any possible "tailing"?
2. Do you wish to avoid contamination with previous samples by only using the separation system once?

3. Do you wish to choose from a maximum possible number of solvents for your substance, since the solvent evaporates completely before the actual separation?

4. Do you wish to choose from a wide range of commercially available stationary phases, which you can easily modify?

5. Do you wish to optimize your separation fast and at low cost by straightforward change of mobile and stationary phase?

6. Do you wish to subject a chromatogram to another chromatographic run at right angles to the first direction, and thus improve the separation (two-dimensional TLC)?

7. Are you looking for a screening method (test procedure for pre-selection of suitable separation systems) which can be transferred to a thicker bed or column for preparative applications?

8. Do you wish to separate as many samples as possible simultaneously and thus save time and money and also co-chromatograph standard substances under identical conditions?

9. Do you wish to have a choice of a maximum possible number of detection systems, possibly in series, and in the case of UV detection wish to purchase just one detector for several chromatographic workplaces (detection of the finished chromatogram can generally wait)?

10. Do you wish to use a simple detection method valid for numerous substances (fluorescence quenching)?

Of course, the question whether TLC is better than other methods does not arise. TLC and column chromatography are complementary methods. TLC is very suited for beginners, for training laboratories, for rapid checks on the course of a synthesis, for checking on drugs at pharmacies. More rigorous demands on separating power and repeatability are met by commercially available high performance systems (HPTLC), sample application devices, developing chambers, and detectors, all of which compare well with other methods. However, certain minimum amount of basic knowledge and practical experience is needed to profitably use TLC as there are several factors which can influence separation in this "open chromatographic system".

Method development for TLC

1. Set your analytical objectives—qualitative identification or quantitative.
2. Separation of two components or multi-component mixtures.
3. Collect information about the sample : structure, polarity, solubility and volatility.

Plates

Hand-made plates : The amount of each sorbent indicated is sufficient to coat five plates of 20 × 20 cm each.

1. *Cellulose (native) :* To 15 g of native fibrous cellulose, add about 100 ml of distilled water, mix with an electric stirrer for 1 min to produce a homogeneous slurry. Spread the slurry with an applicator set at 250 µm. Allow to dry the plates in air and then dry at 110°C for 15 mins.

Note : Amount of water can be varied depending upon the thickness of slurry.

2. *Cellulose with starch as binder :* Suspend 0.4 g of starch in about 10 ml of water, pour the suspension into 90 ml of boiling water. Boil the suspension for 60 s, add 20 g

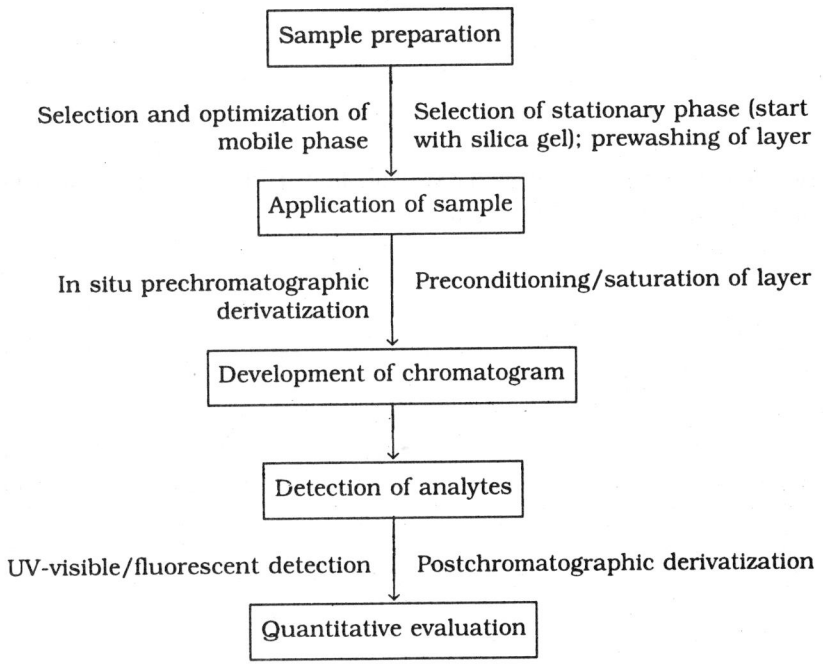

of acid-washed cellulose. Homogenize the slurry with the help of electric stirrer (30 s). Plates are immediately coated while the slurry is still hot. Allow to dry the plates in air or by heating at 110°C for 45 mins. Activation at elevated temperature is avoided. Usual layer thickness so obtained is 200 µm.

3. *Cellulose (microcrystalline)* : Suspend 20 g of cellulose (microcrystalline) in 60 ml of water. Stir in an electric mixture exactly for 30 s to homogenize the slurry. Plates are coated with spreader. Dry the plates in air or by heating at 110°C for 30 mins. No activation at elevated temperature is required. Layer thickness is about 100 µm.

Note : If the slurry is stirred longer than 30 s, swollen condition of the powder is changed resulting in increase in development time of the so prepared plates.

4. *Cellulose (microcrystalline) with fluorescent indicator* : Suspend 25 g of cellulose (microcrystalline) in 40 ml of methanol (this will ensure uniform distribution of indicator), add 20 ml of water, homogenize in electric stirrer exactly for 30 s. The plates so prepared are dried in the air or by heating at 110°C for 30 min. No activation is necessary at elevated temperature. Layer thickness is about 100 µm.

5. *Acelytated cellulose + $CaSO_4 \cdot \frac{1}{2}H_2O$* : Suspend 30 g of acelytated cellulose and 4.5 g of $CaSO_4$ in a mixture containing 60 ml of water and 10 ml of methanol. Stir in an electric stirrer for 30 s to get homogeneous slurry. Sometime air bubbles get trapped which can be removed by pouring 2-3 ml of methanol over slurry, followed by shaking. Use the slurry thus prepared within 10 min for coating the plates. Dry the coated plates in air or by heating at 110°C for 30 min, layer thickness is about 130 µm.

6. *Silica gel or silica gel G* : Suspend 30 g of silica gel or silica gel G in 60-65 ml of water, mix in an electric stirrer to get homogeneous slurry. The plates so coated may be dried in air or by heating for 45 min at 110°C. In case of silica gel G, the slurry must be

used within 2 min. Activation of plates can be carried out by heating at 110°C for 30 min. Layer thickness is usually 250 μm.

7. *Silica gel with starch* : 30 g of silica gel (starch) is suspended in 90 ml of boiling water, homogenized, spread while still hot. Dry the plates in air or by heating at 110°C for 45 min. For activation of the plates, heating at 110°C for 30 min is adequate. Usual layer thickness is 250 μm.

***Precoated plates* :** With the availability of precoated plates commercially, the use of laboratory hand-made plates is on decline. The precoated plates with different support material (glass, aluminium, plastic) and with different sorbent layers are available in different format and thickness by various manufacturers [Merck, Germany; Whatman International Ltd., England; Macherey-Nagel (M & N), Germany; Schleicher & Schuell, Germany]. Usually plates with sorbent thickness of 100-250 μm are used for qualitative and quantitative analysis. However, for preparative TLC work, plates with sorbent thickness of 1.0 - 2.0 mm are available in addition to chemically modified layers.

***Glass support* :** It is resistant to heat and chemicals, easy to handle and always offers superior flat and smooth surface for chromatographic work; disadvantage being fragility, relativity high weight (plate is usually 1.3 mm thick), additional packing material and higher production cost. The precoated plates with glass support are therefore most expensive ready to use layers.

***Polyester (plastic) sheets (0.2 mm thick)* :** More economical as they are produced even in roll forms, unbreakable, less packing material, less shelf space for storage, can be cut to any required format. Spots can be cut and eluted, thus eliminating dust of scrapping. Charring reactions are possible but temperature should not exceed 120°C as the plates are dimensionally unstable (lose shape) beyond this temperature.

***Aluminium sheet (0.1 mm thick)* :** Aluminium sheets as support offer the same advantage as polyester support but with increased temperature resistance. However with eluents containing high concentration of mineral acids or concentrated ammonia, one may find problem as they will chemically attack aluminium. Aluminium sheets are otherwise compatible with organic solvents and organic acids such as formic acid and acetic acid.

Code Letters and Numbers Used in Product Designation

G = Gypsum ($CaSO_4 \cdot \frac{1}{2}H_2O$) used as a binder (layers containing gypsum as binder are loose and suitable for preparative chromatography involving scrapping and elution)

S = Starch, used as a binder (not suitable for detection with iodine)

O = Organic binder (polymeric organic compounds); organic binders impart mechanical strength, durability and abrasion resistance to layers, hence least damaged during shipping and handling

H = Containing no foreign binder

R = Specially purified layers

W = Wettable layers; water tolerant

F = Layers containing fluorescent indicators

$F_{254 + 366}$ = Fluorescent indicators with respective excitation wavelengths

P = Layers for preparative chromatography (thickness 1-2 mm)

F_{254s} = Layers with acid stable fluorescent indicator that is stimulated to pale blue fluorescence on emission at 254 nm, usually used in reversed-phase layers

C = Chanelled layers (layers divided into lanes), prevents cross–contamination while separating multiple samples

RP = Reversed–phase

RP_2 , RP_8 and RP_{18} = Reversed–phase with C_2 , C_8 or C_{18} hydrocarbon chain

NH_2 = Hydrophilic layers with amino modification

CN = Hydrophilic layers with cyano modification

CHIR = Chiral layers for separation of optically active isomers based on ligand exchange

DIOL = Hydrophilic layers with DIOL modification

Commonly available precoated plates with their applications

1. Silica gel 60F (unmodified) : More than 80% analysis are done on this layer. This layer is available with suitable indicator (adsorption and partition chromatography).
2. Aluminium oxide : Basic substances, alkaloids and steroids.
3. High purity silica gel 60 : Aflotoxins
4. Cellulose (microcrystalline) : Amino acid, dipeptides, sugars, antibiotics and other labile compounds which cannot be chromatographed on active layers of silica gel.
5. PEI impregnated cellulose : Mono and oligonucleotides, co-enzymes, sugar phosphate.
6. Polymide/micropolymide : Dansyl-amino acids, anti-oxidants, anti-pyretics, optical brightners, dyestuffs, pesticides, porphyrins, steroids, hormones, vitamins, sulphonamides, sugars.
7. Silica gel, chemically modified (Fig. 1).
   (a) NH_2 (amino) : Carboxylic acid, phenols, nucleotides, vitamins (B_1, B_6, B_{12}), uric acid, xanthine derivatives.
   (b) CN (cyano) : Pharmaceutical preservatives.
   (c) CHIR : Resolution of enantiomeric substances for optical purity such as amino acids, dipeptides, lactones. These plates are coated with reversed-phase silica gel and then impregnated with a chiral selector (a proline derivative) and copper (++) ion. The separation of optical isomers is based on ligand exchange, the chiral selector (on the plate) and enantiomer to be separated. The mixed chelate-complex with transition element (Cu^{++}) have different stabilities which results in chromatographic separation. For optimal separation and reproducibility of Rf values, activation prior to spotting (100°C for 15 min) and chamber saturation may be required. Application of chiral plate in separation of amino acids, dipeptides, lactones has been reported by Nyiredy et al.
   (d) DIOL : Hormones, steroids.
   (e) Impregnated plates : Plates impregnated with liquid paraffin, buffers, silver nitrate (shelf life is limited), ion-exchange material, acid, bases, or detergents.
   (f) RP-2, RP-8 and RP-18 : Non-polar substances (lipids), fatty acids, carotenoids, steroids, cholesterol and its esters. Polar substances, basic and acidic drugs

which are likely to decompose on active layers, vitamins, antibiotics, amino acids, chloroplast pigments, phenothiazine tranquilizers, cannabinoids, preservatives, sulphonamides, insecticides (DDT, endrin, aldrin), alkaloids (ephedrine, atropine, scopolamine, codeine, morphine), barbiturates, analgesics, cardiac drugs, sweeteners, food dyes, tranquilizers, anti-oxidants.

Note : Chemical reaction of the polar silanol group of silica gel with alkylsilanes of different chain lengths yields reversed-phases. Hydrophobic character increases with increasing chain lengths of hydrocarbon. Low degree of modification means weak interaction between the sample molecule and the stationary phase, thus leading to higher Rf values as HPTLC plates with silica gel 60RP-18W with low degree of modification show higher Rf value than HPTLC with RP-18 modification.

8. Prescored : 20 × 20 cm precoated glass plate has three scored marks, can be snapped up.

9. Preparatory plates : Layer thickness of 1 - 2 mm, large sample volumes can be applied as streak. These are usually available as precoated soft layers, to be used when separated substances are to be recovered, usually gives less sample resolution than analytical plates. These plates are preferred to column chromatography due to ease in recovery of separated zones, sample volume should be moderate.

10. Hybrid plates (RP18WF$_{254s}$) : These plates are suitable both for reversed-phase and normal-phase chromatography. They can be developed using aqueous mobile phases as well as mixture of aqueous-organic solvents. HPTLC grade silica gel 60 (mean pore size 6 nm) forms the basis for these plates. Controlled reaction conditions ensure that certain portion of available silanol groups are chemically bonded with octadecyl chain whereas the remaining silanol groups remain non-bonded, thus giving hybrid (hydrophobic and hydrophilic) character to the plates. Conventional reversed-phase plates resist the flow of the eluent considerably and sometime completely depending on the proportion of water present in the mobile phase. To avoid this limitation, the partial chemical bonding of silanol groups results in hybrid nature of the plate, which makes the plates wettable (W) depending on the residual hydrophilicity of layer. In such plates, the development time is significantly reduced for strongly polar eluents. As untreated silanol groups are blocked by the water in the eluent, this type of incompletely silanized RP coating along with high water contents reversed phase eluents, demonstrates strong reversed-phase characteristics as compared to fully silanized RP layers, conventionally used. Such hybrid plates have application in chromatographic separation of preser- vatives, barbiturates, analgesics, phenothiazines, amino acids and flavonoids.

11. Prescreen TLC plates : RPTLC C18 plates in the size of 5 × 7.5 cm are available for quick and inexpensive preview of separation traits prior to HPLC analysis. This can be of help in optimizing sample preparation parameters for use in HPLC.

12. Plates with preabsorbent layer (concentration zone) : Sample enrichment by evaporation while applying the sample can accommodate large volumes, hence less need to concentrate dilute sample solutions.

13. Dual-phase TLC plates : Part of the plate is coated with reversed-phase layer, while the remaining has normal phase coating.

Plate size

Precoated TLC/HPTLC plates in size of 20 × 20 cm with aluminium or polyester support are usually procured mainly for economic reasons. These plates can be cut to size and

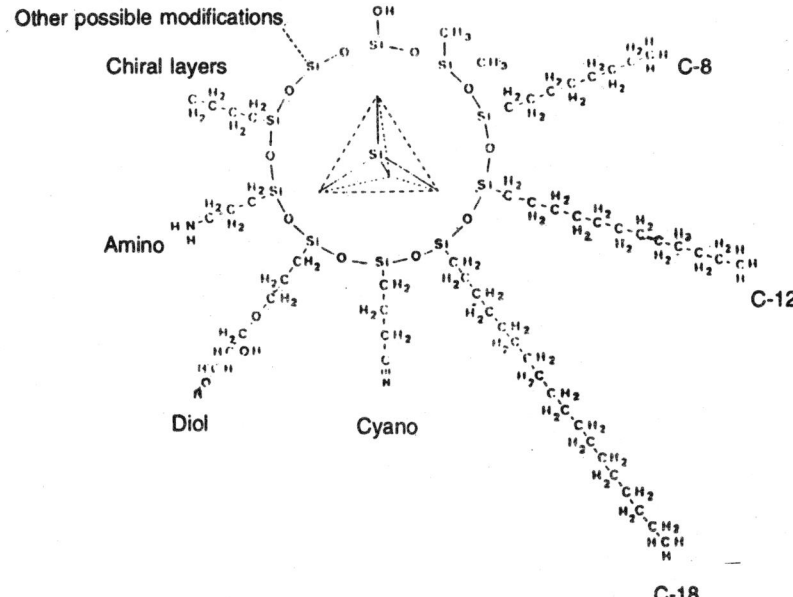

Fig. 1. Chemically modified silica gel layers (CN, NH₂, Diol, C-2, C-8, C-12, C-18 and Chiral). *Courtesy :* E. Merck (India) Ltd.

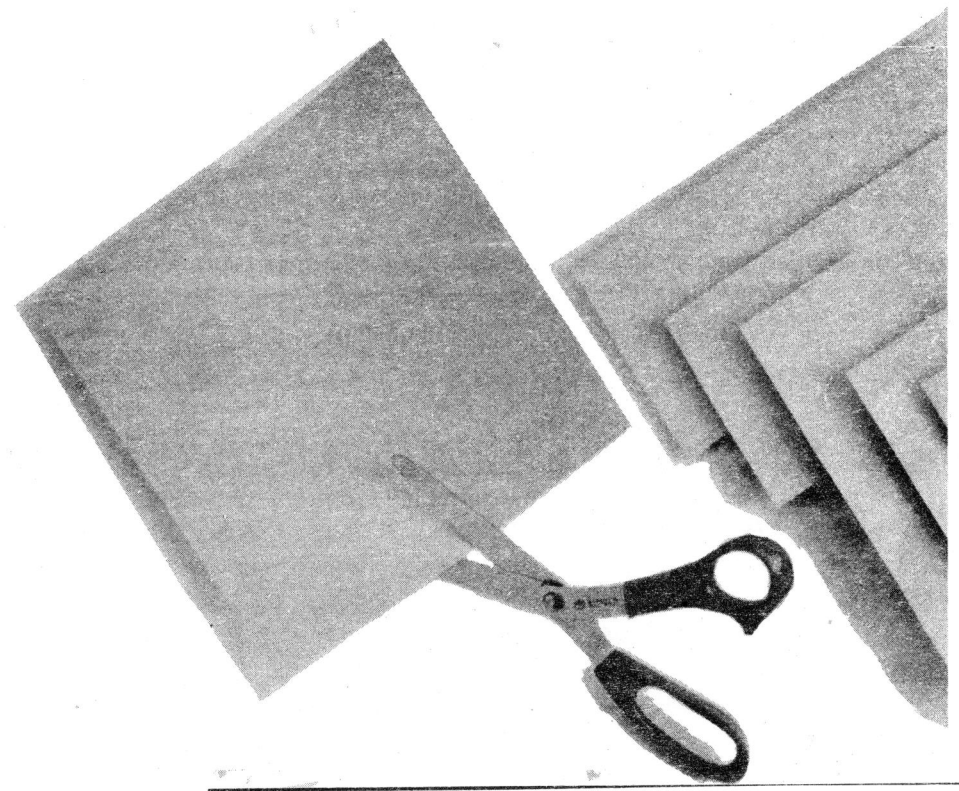

Fig. 2. Inclination of scissors blades for proper cutting of a TLC plate of a particular size.

shape (format) to suit particular analysis by using general purpose scissors. Before handling the precoated plates for any experimental work, it is important to note direction of the application of sorbent as chromatographic developments have to be/must be performed in that direction only. Good cut edges are obtained if the scissors blades are sharp. Scissors blades should always be inclined slightly to the right (Fig. 2). Any layer which has been loosened as a result of cut should be removed by lightly drawing the spatula over the cut edge. This is necessary to obtain constant Rf values over the entire width of the layer. Scissors blades if inclined to the left leads to flaking off of the layer on one or both sides of the cut. This will result in the formation of capillary cracks between the chromatographic layer and the foil in which mobile phase will travel much more rapidly forward than it does in the centre of the chromatogram. Such cracks will also cause mobile phase to migrate from edges of the layer to the centre thus causing deformation of zones and distortion of tracks.

Prewashing of precoated plates

Sorbents with large surface area absorb not only water vapours and other impurities from atmosphere but other volatile substances often condense particularly after the packing has been opened and exposed to laboratory atmosphere for a long time. Such impurities including elutable components of the binder usually give dirty zones and fail to give reproducible results. It is only for these reasons that precoated plates are always packed with the glass or foil side upward (coated layer downward). To avoid any possible interference due to impurities with the chromatographic separation particularly in case of quantitative work, it is always recommended to clear the plates before actual chromato- graphy. This process is called prewashing of plates. Ascending, dipping, continuous mode are the common methods of cleaning the plates. Ascending (blank chromatography) technique takes somewhat longer time but cleaning effect is superior, however, active dirt gets accumulated at solvent front. Therefore compounds of interest that migrate at the rear end of solvent front are partially obscured by overlapping fluorescence of the surface contaminants. Thus compounds with HRf value of 75 and above will be difficult to scan particularly under fluorescent mode. This difficulty is often overcome by cutting 10-20% of the upper portion of prewashed plate before proceeding with chromatographic separation.

The other most commonly employed method for prewashing is dipping. Quicker dipping process yields rather uniform clean layer but cleaning effect is often not as good as with ascending technique. Maxwell et al., 1990, have suggested the use of specially designed chambers designated as A, B, C, each containing about 10 ml of the cleaning solvent. For prewashing, the plates are first dipped into chamber marked 'A' for one minute, then taken to chamber 'B'. The chamber can easily clean 20 plates (10 × 10 cm). After initial cleaning process, the chamber marked 'A' is rejected and chamber 'B' serves as initial cleaning chamber, while chamber 'C' is used for secondary cleaning.

Excellent results are obtained if the plates are subjected to prewashing by continuous mode for some time, i.e., in a chamber closed by a lid having a slit.

After washing, the plates must be dried for a sufficient time to ensure complete removal of the washing liquids (usually for methanol 30-60 min at 105° are required). Use of hot or cold air (hair drier) should be avoided as laboratory air which is usually contaminated is blown over the layer and purpose of cleaning the layer is defeated. The washed plates should always be stored in a dust-free atmosphere under ambient conditions. Preferably desiccators of suitable dimensions should be used for storing both cleaned and uncleaned plates. No grease should be used for sealing the desiccator. Use of drying agents is also not necessary.

Prewashing of plates must be done to at least 1-2 cm longer than the subsequent actual chromatographic development so that any dirt accumulated at the front does not interfere in densitometric scanning. As a result of prewashing, signal to noise ratio' is substantially low and base lines are straighter, both these steps essential for quantitative analysis by in situ densitometry. Reduction in signal to noise ratio as a result of prewashing improves the limit of detection (LOD) of the procedure.

Note : As after prewashing, activation of the layer in drying cup-board to remove the washing solvent is essential, analysts often experience difficulty in drying aluminium-backed layers as the foil tends to lose shape during drying/activation. Obviously any distortion of the layer will make remaining steps of separation more difficult and often impossible. It is, therefore, suggested that aluminium-backed precoated plates should be dried by keeping it between two blank glass plates.

Even for routine analysis (qualitative), one must use prewashed plates, otherwise, the dirt front will interfere in the detection of substances with high Rf values, i.e., more than 70. Methanol is the most commonly employed solvent for prewashing but its cleaning power is not good particularly when lipophilic mobile phases are to be used for subsequent chromatographic development. In such cases, it is preferable to carry out prewashing process with mobile phase in question. However, mobile phase containing acid or alkali should be avoided as they may not be completely removed during subsequent activation, thus impregnating the stationary phase. Mixtures of chloroform in methanol (1 : 1); ethyl acetate–methanol (1 : 1); chloroform–methanol–ammonia (90 : 10 : 1) have been used as solvents for prewashing. Methylene chloride–methanol (1 : 1) is best suited for removing any impurity picked up during storage in laboratory atmosphere. One may also try prewashing with 1% ammonia solution or 1% acetic acid in methanol.

Activation of precoated plates

Freshly opened box of TLC/HPTLC plates usually does not require activation. However, plates exposed to high humidity or kept on hand for long time may have to be activated by placing in oven at 110-120°C for 30 minutes prior to sample spotting (aluminium-backed plates should be activated by keeping between two glass plates). This step removes water that has been physically absorbed on the surface of the sorbent. After the plates are removed from prewash chambers, they should always be dried in vertical position as in horizontal position drops of solvent may fall on the plate as a result of condensation. Activation at higher temperature and for longer time should be avoided as it may lead to very active layers and there will be risk of samples being decomposed or artifact being formed. In such cases, it is advisable to resort to use of RPTLC plates.

Note : As application of sample(s) usually takes several minutes, the activity of the solvent layer even after activation is likely to correspond to the relative humidity of the experimental room. Prior activation may therefore not be required as layer in fact adapts to the relative humidity of the room. An air-conditioned room with air lock system is usually effective in maintaining the humidity and temperature at reasonably constant level.

Sample preparation

The sample preparation is not as demanding as for other chromatographic techniques, however, several steps for sample pretreatment may be necessary such as sampling, mechanical crushing, extraction, filtration and enrichment of minor compounds. Proper sample preparation is an important prerequisite for success of thin layer chromatographic separation. The sample preparation procedure is to dissolve the dosage form with complete recovery of intact compound(s) of interest and minimum of matrix with a suitable concentration of analyte(s) for direct application on the HPTLC plate. Besides maximizing the yield of analytes in the selected solvent, stability of analytes during extraction and analysis must be considered and ensured. Therefore, the choice of a suitable solvent for a given analysis is very important. For normal phase chromatography using silica gel precoated plates (more than 80-90% of TLC analysis is done using silica gel as sorbent), solvent for dissolving the sample should be non-polar and volatile as far as possible, since polar solvents are likely to induce circular chromatography at origin, particularly when sample is applied in increment on top of each other, leading to spreading of spot, thus loss of separation efficiency. For reversed-phase chromatography, usually polar solvents are used for dissolving the sample, however, such polar solvents must wet the sorbent so that sample penetrates the layer uniformly.

Clean-up steps in the sample preparation, if necessary, must be optimized. Sufficient quantity of sample should be initially taken for clean-up steps. Once the sample is cleaned up, one must ensure that it is subjected to chromatographic separation as quickly as possible particularly while dealing with labile substances, storage, if necessary, should only be in refrigerator.

It is preferable to keep the solvent as simple as possible and quantity employed be limited to ensure complete extraction of analytes and minimum of extraneous component. Sample and reference substances should be dissolved in the same solvent to ensure comparable distribution at starting zones.

Choice of solvent for the sample

- It should dissolve the analytes.
- Should be reasonably volatile.
- Should have low viscosity.
- Wets the sorbent layer.
- Should be a weak chromatographic solvent for the analyte.

For TLC on silica gel, the use of weakest (least polar) solvent which allows quantitative dissolving and spotting of sample and there is no preliminary development and separation within the initial spot at the origin, is recommended (Fig. 3). Rf values of the components of the interest in the selected solvent for preparation of the sample should be less than 0.1%.

Evaporation of solvent

Whenever sample requires concentration, use of rotary evaporator with attached round bottom flask is recommended. The solution should be first evaporated completely to dryness and then the residue is dissolved in same or different solvent for application to the TLC layer. Use of non-polar solvent to dissolve the residue will help to remove polar impurities which will remain undissolved. Solvents with high boiling point or polarity are difficult to remove solvent layers during application. If a small amount of solvent is left after application, it can cause serious effects on the separation by causing zone spreading or deformation. Use of hot air to dry the solvent at origin should normally be discouraged

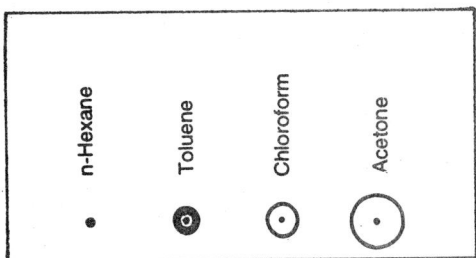

Fig. 3. Influence of solvent on the size of sample zone.

as it can cause decomposition of heat labile substances on the surface of an active sorbent.

Application of sample

Sample application is the most critical step for obtaining good resolution. The sample should be completely transferred to the layer, however, under no circumstances, the application process should damage the layer, as damaged layer results in unevenly shaped spots. Wherever possible, use of automatic application devices is recommended for quantitative analysis. While using graduated capillaries, one must ensure that they fill and empty completely.

The sample should be applied through clean upper end of the capillary and for that after filling the capillary to marked point, reverse the capillary for applying the sample.

Note : Sample solution in high density solvents such as chloroform may leave the capillary before sample application, whereas solutions of high viscosity may incompletely enter or leave the capillaries, high volatile solvents such as acetone, diethyl ether may undergo partial evaporation before application. Under such circumstances, the use of microsyringe is recommended if laboratory is not equipped with automatic application devices.

Usually application of 1-10 µl volume for TLC and 0.5-5 µl for HPTLC is recommended keeping the size of starting zone(s) down to minimum; 2-4 mm (TLC) and 0.5-1 mm (HPTLC) in the concentration range of 0.1-1 µg/µl for TLC/HPTLC. Substance zones which are too large from the beginning cause poor separation as during development spots do tend to become large and more diffused. This difficulty is more pronounced in case of substances with high Rf values. It is therefore recommended that solution should be applied in small increments with intermediate drying (use cold or hot air or nitrogen in case of labile compounds, asymmetric accelerated evaporation of the solvent from the point of application can lead to local changes in the concentration in spotted substances) particularly when the sample solution is predominantly aqueous.

Note : Application in small increments has disadvantage as well, since previously applied zones may get chromatographed on each subsequent application leading to formation of horse-shoe shaped developed spot. For application, sample and reference solutions should possibly contain the same matrix, otherwise matrix present in the sample can cause changes in Rf values.

However, volume and concentration primarily depend on the component under analysis and their sensitivity to various detection techniques. If too much sample is applied, it may not be absorbed uniformly throughout the layer leading to overloading, as a result trailing of zones and poor resolution is observed. Problem arising out of such overloading when unavoidable, can best be overcome by applying the sample as band, the only apparent disadvantage being that only fewer samples can be accommodated on a given plate.

Advantages of application of sample as band are :

- Better separation because of rectangular area in which the compounds are present on the plate.
- Equal Rf values of the compounds from sample and reference solution.
- Matrix effect of extracted and applied excipients are significantly reduced as solution is distributed over a larger area.
- Response of densitometer is higher than observed from an equal amount/equal volume of the same solution applied as a spot. It appears that light may not gain access to all the sample material applied as a spot (point). This is supported by the observation that range of linearity is small for pointwise application than for bandwise application.
- Application of different volumes as bands from one solution gives same concentration-response curve as obtained by application of equal volumes of solution with different concentration. This correlation is absent when sample solution is applied as a spot. This is significant as while preparing the concentration-response curve, one need not prepare solutions with different concentration while applying the sample as a band.
- Generally speaking, spot broadening in the direction of development is smaller in the case of bandwise application.
- Larger quantities of the sample can be handled for application, thus reducing the need for concentration step which may be quite damaging in case of labile substances.
- Position of plate for densitometric scanning is less critical as composition of the compounds is uniform in the entire area of band.

Note : It is recommended that samples should not be applied on outer (both) edges of the plate (leave at least 1-2 mm on each side) as rate of solvent evaporation is usually greater at the edges than near the centre of the plate. Rf value is greater near the edges due to boundary/edge effect.

Mobile phase (MP)

Poor grade of solvent used in preparing mobile phases have been found to decrease resolution, spot definition and Rf reproducibility. Mobile phase commonly called solvent system is traditionally selected by controlled process of trial and error and also based on one's own experience in the field. It is often possible that few layer-solvent combinations already reported in the literature for compounds of interest or similar compounds may be suitable in a given analytical problem with minor modifications. Nevertheless, it should not be forgotten that such conditions may have been chosen due to availability rather than suitability and often improvements are required. Manufacturers of sorbents and precoated plates usually supply bibliographies of separations that they have carried out in their application laboratories. However, mobile phase should be chosen taking into consideration chemical properties of analytes and the sorbent layer. Use of mobile phase containing more than three or four components should normally be avoided as it is often difficult to get reproducible ratios of different components.

- Solvent composition is expressed by volumes (v/v) and usually sum of total volume is 100.
- Various components of MP should be measured separately and then placed in the

mixing vessel. This will not only prevent the contamination of solvent stock by evaporation from already partially filled mixing vessel but also any possible volumetric error arising due to volumes expansion (dilation) or contraction on mixing.

- Laboratories equipped with complete HPTLC system usually use smaller development chamber such as twin trough chambers (10 × 10 cm) where comparatively smaller volumes of MP usually 10-15 ml is required. It is advisable that different components of the MP should be measured with volumetric pipettes.
- Different components of MP should be first mixed in mixing vessel and then introduced into the developing chamber.
- Chambers usually containing multi-component mobile phase once used is not recommended for re-use for any future development work as composition of MP is likely to change during chromatographic development, due to differential evaporation and adsorption by the layer and also once the chamber is opened, each solvent component will evaporate disproportionately depending on their volatilities.
- Solvent components which are relatively volatile at room temperature and may play significant role in final MP such as pH of the solvent system should not be used for long time after the container is once opened, such as strong solution of ammonia, glacial acetic acid or diethylamine.
- Chemical reaction may occur between different components of MP such as acetic acid and ammonia.
- Polar solvent portion of MP may get adsorbed by the layer during development.
- In bi-component MP loss of more volatile minor component such as ammonia is worth considering.
- Mobile phase should be as simple as possible and permissible by analytes and sample matrix.
- Some form of MP optimization is generally necessary when performing HPTLC. (Mobile phase selection and optimization has been reviewed by Nurok, 1989.)

Optimization of mobile phase (solvent optimization)

First level : Neat solvents from different selectivity area were tested. Within a selectivity area solvents may give similar separation. Usually diethylether, ethanol, methanol, tetrahydrofuran, dimethyl formamide, dichloromethane, ethylacetate, acetonitrite, methylethyl ketone, toluene and chloroform are used as neat solvents.

If acceptable resolution and medium Rf range is achieved, the analyst can directly try level 3, i.e., exploring the suitability of solvent mixture. However, if level 1 does not yield satisfactory results, then proceed with level 2.

Second level : From level 1, solvents which leave the main fraction/component of the analyte near the starting point or close to the solvent front, are required to be adjusted in strength. If Rf values are too high, solvent strength should be decreased by adding non-polar solvents such as n-hexane, toluene. If Rf values are too low, the solvent strength is required to be increased by addition of methanol, ethanol or water. In such case, usual ratio of 9 : 1, 8 : 2, 7 : 3, 6 : 4, 5 : 5 are tried.

Third level : Mixtures of solvents from different selectivity group are investigated; the strength is adjusted, if necessary. These solvent mixtures can be binary, tertiary or even quaternary. Usually one should start with the centre and corner position of selectivity such as in the case of binary mixtures, the ratios are 1 : 1, 9 : 1, 1 : 9, and for tertiary mixtures 1 : 1 : 1, 8 : 1 : 1 and 1 : 1 : 8 ratios should be first tried.

At this level, addition of small amount of acidic (acetic acid) or basic (triethylamine) modifiers significantly enhance the separation efficiency of mobile phase.

Fourth level : At this level, final optimization of the mobile phase to be used for a particular separation is made. To get the best separation, small variations in the proportions of different solvents may have to be made.

A simple spot test (Fig. 4) can be extremely useful indicator for selection of solvent. The solution of the analyte to be separated is spotted at several different places on the layer of desired sorbent. Then tip of the capillary filled with mobile phase (solvent) is placed in the middle of each applied spot. Due to capillary action, the solvent leaving the capillary spreads in circular fashion and may separate the analyte like a circular chromatogram. Comparison of these results can provide definite guide for selection of mobile phase and the sorbent.

Caution

Use of multicomponent mobile phases which are partially miscible : Use of upper or lower layer of partially miscible solvent mixtures as mobile phases can lead to severe disturbances during development of chromatogram because, as soon as there is slight change in temperature, the pure and homogeneous upper or lower phase initially employed generally separates into new two-phase system with each of the two newly formed phases having a different composition. This is however frequently not noticed on account of small volume (few drops). On account of difference in composition from main body of M.P., these few drops of M.P. can cause considerable disturbances particularly when they float to the top and are preferentially taken up onto the TLC layer. These behave as circular barrier for M.P. that stream pass them.

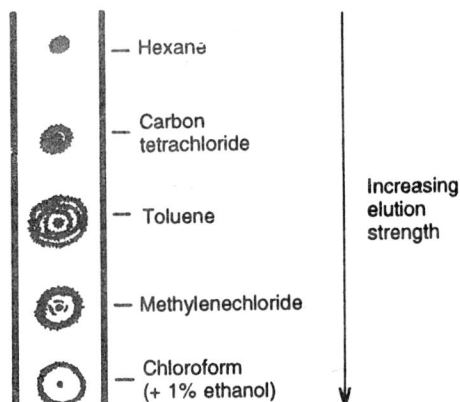

Fig. 4. Spot test for determination of suitable solvent for chromatography.

Preconditioning (Chamber saturation)

Chamber saturation has pronounced influence on the separation profile. When the plate is introduced into an unsaturated chamber (Fig. 5A), during the course of development, the solvent evaporates from the plate mainly at the solvent front. Therefore larger quantity of the solvent shall be required for a given distance, hence resulting is increase in Rf values. If the tank is saturated (by lining with filter paper) prior to development (Fig. 5B), solvent vapours soon get uniformly distributed throughout the chamber. As soon as the plate is placed in such a saturated chamber, it soon gets preloaded with solvent vapours, hence less solvent shall be required to travel a particular distance, resulting in lower Rf values.

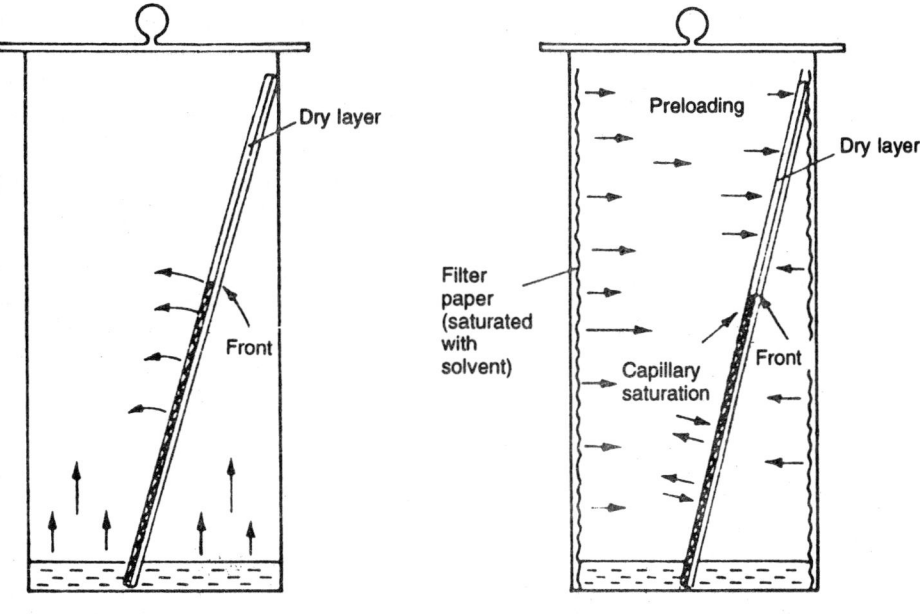

A. Unsaturated chamber   **. B.** Saturated chamber

Fig. 5. Influence of vapour phase on the development of chromatograms.

Note : Time required for saturation will depend on the nature and composition of mobile phase and layer thickness (equilibrating time increases with increase in layer thickness).

While dealing with solvent of low polarity such as aliphatic hydrocarbons; toluene and their mixtures, the preloading of dry layer with solvent vapours should be avoided. However, preequilibrium is often recommended in case of solvent with high polarity such as methanol. Development in a non-saturated or partially saturated atmosphere is recommended with solvents used in a composition leading to phase separation such as mixture of n-butanol, water, glacial acetic acid. However in case of RPTLC, it is always preferable to saturate the chamber with methanol as normally in RPTLC, MP with high water contents are employed. If chromatographic procedure is to be carried out at a controlled relative humidity of the chamber, then suitable liquid is placed in one of the troughs of twin-trough chamber. Usually relative humidity of the room in controlled by dehumidifier. However, if experiments are required to be carried at specific RH, then solution of sulphuric acid or salt solutions may be employed.

Development and drying

Ascending, descending, two-dimensional, horizontal, multiple overrun (continuous), gradient, radial (circular), anti-radial (anti-circular), multimodal (multi-dimensional), forced flow planar chromatography are the most common modes of chromatographic development. Rectangular glass chambers, twin-trough chambers, V-shaped chambers, sandwich chambers, horizontal development chambers, vario-KS chambers, circular and anti-circular, U chambers and automated multiple development chambers are commonly used for carrying out different types of TLC development.

Note : Under no circumstances, develop the chromatogram until and unless solvent of the applied sample is completely evaporated—it usually takes 5-10 minutes.

Since HPTLC is now a well accepted analytical technique for quantitative analysis, reagents often used for detection should no longer merely be visualized for identification only but should be expected to give reproducible and stoichiometric reactions suitable for quantitative analysis. It is therefore, important that once the chromatogram is developed, it should be handled with utmost care. Application of reagents if required has to be homogeneous ensuring uniform reaction and finally stabilizing of end reaction product.

After development the plate is removed from the chamber and MP is removed as completely and as quickly as possible. This step should preferably be performed in fume cup board to avoid contamination of laboratory atmosphere. The plates should always be laid horizontally so that while MP evaporates the separated substances will migrate evenly to the surface where they can be easily detected.

Usually analysts may employ hand dryer (hot or cold) to effect faster removal of the mobile phase, however following needs consideration :

- Essential oil components may evaporate.
- Compounds sensitive to oxygen may get destroyed due to rise in temperature while using hot air dryer.
- Particles of dust from laboratory may deposit on the chromatogram which may influence the ultimate densitometric scanning.
- Chemical vapours present in the laboratory are likely to be transported in the air stream onto the layer. This will positively interfere when postchromatographic derivatization is resorted to.

It is precisely for these reasons that drying of chromatogram should preferably be done in vacuum desiccator with protection from heat and light.

Factors/parameters influencing the TLC separation and resolution of spots

1. Type of stationary phase (sorbent), its particle size and activity.
2. Type of plates (precoated or hand-made).
3. Layer thickness (any deviation in layer thickness).
4. pH of the layer.
5. Binder in the layer.
6. Mobile phase (solvent system).
7. Solvent purity.
8. Type and size of developing chamber.
9. Degree of chamber saturation.
10. Solvent for the sample preparation.
11. Sample volume spotted.
12. Size (diameter) of the initial spot.
13. Solvent/mobile phase level in the chamber.
14. Distance between starting zone and level of eluent in the chamber.
15. Gradient.
16. Relative humidity.
17. Temperature (Rf values usually increase with the rise in temperature).
18. Flow rate of the solvent, velocity of mobile phase.
19. Separation distance.
20. Mode of development.

Greater the distance between different spots and smaller the initial spot diameter of the sample, better the resolution.

While describing the result of any TLC/HPTLC procedure, various parameters and conditions under which results for a specific analysis have been obtained must be documented. This is absolutely essential for possible reproducible results.

Note : In daily practice, one can either rely upon his own experience or gained from other sources, or one can survey the literature to retrieve the information and then optimise.

Evaluation of a thin layer chromatogram

The evaluation depends on the purpose of a chromatographic analysis. For qualitative determination often localization of substances is sufficient. This can be easily achieved by parallel runs with reference substances.

Rf values

A parameter often used for qualitative evaluation is the Rf value (retention factor) or the 100-fold value hRf. The Rf value (Fig. 6) is defined as follows :

$$Rf = \frac{\text{Distance starting line–middle of spot}}{\text{Distance starting line–solvent front}} = \frac{b}{a}$$

i.e. Rf values are between 0 and 1, best between 0.1 and 0.8 (i.e. 10-80 for hRf).

The distance travelled by a substance should be measured from the centre of the spots which are round but spots showing tailing, the measurement is done from the middle of most dense areas. As the Rf values are likely to be affected by numbers of factors, it is desirable that the authentic sample and the drug under analysis should be run simultaneously on the same plate. This is the procedure usually used for pharmacopoeial purposes.

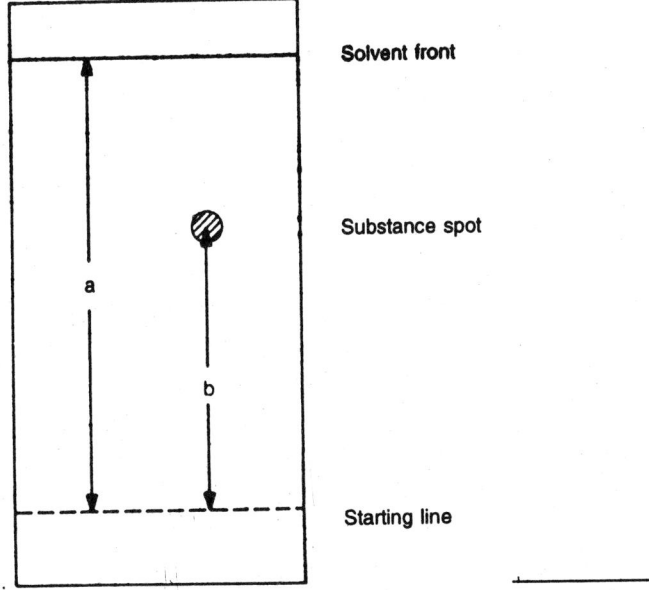

Fig. 6. Measurement of distance for calculation of Rf values in a developed chromatogram.

If reproducible Rf values are to be obtained, it is, however, essential that several parameters such as chamber saturation, constant composition of solvent mixtures, constant temperature etc. are strictly controlled.

1. *Stationary phase* : The quality of adsorbent, binder, impurity present, uniformity of the plate and degree of activation should be similar on each occasion.

2. *Mobile phase* : This should be prepared accurately from pure grade of solvents and made freshly in case of very volatile solvents.

3. *Development chamber* : Saturation conditions are required to be attained for running TLC plates. This can be accomplished simply by using the smallest possible chamber having filter paper lining on three sides and sufficient solvent. Usually 30 minutes are adequate for equilibrium. The lid of the chamber should be made leak-proof by applying grease on the edges, a 500 ml filled bottle can also be kept on the top of the lid to further ensure its proper sealing.

4. *Temperature* : The exact control of temperature is not necessary. However, chamber should be kept away from source of heat and light as increase in temperature will cause quick evaporation of volatile solvents resulting in faster running of solvents. In such circumstances, Rf values are likely to decrease slightly.

5. *Development distance* : There is no hard and fast rule regarding the running distance but it has been observed that there is an apparent increase in Rf values with increase in running distance due to increased evaporation of the solvent from the upper part of the plate. The distance of 10 cm is usually adequate for effective separation, longer distance usually causes diffusion of the spots.

6. *Amount of sample* : If the plate is over-loaded with the sample, usually a tailing spot is obtained. The amount of sample to be applied can be determined experimentally.

7. *Running the plates* : The saturated developing chamber is normally used. It consists of a glass tank which has ground edges at the top to make an airtight seal with the glass cover when coated with grease. The tank is lined with the filter paper on three sides. The size of the jar depends on the size of the TLC plates; for separation on a microscopic slide, smaller jar is used. It is preferable if the jar is supplied with a hole for adding mobile phase. The quantity of the mobile phase should be adequate to cover the bottom of the plate up to a height of 1 cm. The tank is allowed to equilibrate with solvent vapour for at least 30 minutes. The TLC plate is placed in a vertical position in such a manner that the line of application is always above the level of mobile phase. Special racks are available to hold up to five plates at a time and developed simultaneously.

It is conventional to develop plates for a distance of 10 cm which may require up to 2 hours for a viscous mobile phase particularly in winter season. However, running of the plate for shorter distance has advantage i.e. increase is sensitivity (spots do not diffuse) and a saving of material. The major disadvantage being incomplete resolution, about 20% decrease in resolution by decreasing the development distance from 10 cm to 5 cm. It is always preferable to develop the plate for a predetermined distance. Whenever the plate is removed from the chamber the position of the solvent front should be quickly marked before the solvent evaporates from the plates.

Detection and visualization

One of the most characteristic feature of TLC/HPTLC is the possibility to utilize post-chromatographic off-line derivatization. With availability of many visualization reagents, findings can be confirmed which the HPLC is lacking. These visualization reactions, are possible for identification even if the separation is not optimal (in such cases in situ UV spectra gets disturbed due to closer HRf of related substances).

As soon as the development process is complete, the plate is removed from the chamber and dried to remove the mobile phase completely. The zones can be located by various physical, chemical, biological-physiological methods. There is apparently no difficulty in detecting coloured substances or colourless substances absorbing in short-wave ultraviolet (UV) region (254 nm) or with intrinsic fluorescence such as riboflavin, quinine sulphate. The substances which do not have above properties have to be transferred into detectable substances by means of chromogenic or fluorogenic reagents which are more expensive, time-consuming and complicated.

Detection sensitivity depends on the specificity for the reagent employed. Iodine is the universal detection reagent, the detection is usually non-destructive and reversible but certain substances may be altered through non-reversible derivatization such as ethambutol hydrochloride, a totally non-UV absorbing compound forms a UV absorbing complex with iodine through charge transfer. Iodine is the least sensitive reagent. After the plates are exposed to iodine vapours, the compounds can be identified/located by slightly yellow coloured iodine containing spots. Best results are often obtained by dipping the plate in 0.10 to 0.25% solution of iodine in chloroform–methanol (1 : 1). After evaporation of excess iodine, the plate is covered with a glass sheet and four sides may be sealed with tape to prevent further evaporation of iodine from the spots/bands. This technique has been successfully employed by the author for quantitative estimation of certain non-UV absorbing compounds such as dicyclomine hydrochloride, ethambutol hydrochloride by densitometric scanning of the resultant spot/band at 440 nm (detection with iodine is not suitable for layers containing starch as binder). Although detection reagents to be used in gas phase, such as iodine, hydrochloric acid and ammonia vapours give uniform distribution, but dipping as suggested above, is the method of choice for application of the reagent for reproducible results.

Detection under UV light is the first choice and is non-destructive in most of the cases and is commonly employed for densitometric scanning. However, certain drug substances such as steroids and vitamins (D_2, D_3) are highly sensitive and may undergo molecular rearrangement.

Derivatization reactions are essentially required for detection when individual compound does not respond to UV or does not have intrinsic fluorescence. It is not significant whether derivatization is pre- or postchromatographic, however, prechromatographic derivatization not only helps in detection but enhances the selectivity of the mobile phase or may even stabilize the otherwise labile or volatile compounds such as formaldehyde in medicated tooth-pastes, whereas postchromatographic derivatization helps in detection and may also enhance sensitivity. For postchromatographic derivatization, smaller the chromato-graphic zone, greater the concentration of the substance in particular area leading to increase in detection sensitivity. It is therefore desirable that Rf values of the substances in such cases should be as low as possible as with higher Rf values, spot/band gets diffused. Other simple detection method is based on wetting and solubility phenomena. Aluminium oxide, kieselguhr or silica gel are hydrophilic adsorbents. On dipping or spraying the chromatogram with water, lipophilic substances such as steroids, fatty acids, hydrocarbons, dimethyl polysilixane (silicone oil) appear as white (opaque) spot against semi-transparent background as such substances being immiscible with water are not wetted (take up water less than the layer). This wetting effect is more prominent if the plate is fully saturated with water and held against light. The contrast is best immediately after dipping, disappears on drying. Instead of water. one can employ hydrophilic or lipophilic dye solutions for spraying or dipping. In case of hydrophilic dyes such as methylene blue, the background is stained blue whereas non-wetted zone appears as pale while in case of lipophilic dyes, the non-wetted zone appears as deeply coloured against pale background. Fluorescent chemicals are usually employed for detection of lipophilic substances by wetting/non-wetting technique. Rhodamin B, a fluorescent dye has been used for detection of lipophilic substances forming non-wetted zones as the dye will get concentrated on non-wetted zone leading to increased fluorescence when examined under long UV light (365 nm). Other commonly used reagents are phospho-molybdic acid, antimony trichloride or pentachloride, anisaldehyde–sulphuric acid, dimethyl-aminobenzaldehyde in sulphuric acid, fluorescein sodium and pH indicators. These reagents yield sufficient stable coloured spots for quantitative scanning.

Several corrosive reagents have been used for detection of organic compound by charring on heating after spraying.

Note : If heating of the plate, after it is treated with the reagent, is not uniform, there always exists risk of reaction inhomogeneity on the plate. Usually, drying cup board or hot plates are employed. Drying cup board should have non-perforated shelf. Perforated shelf is not suitable as heat transfer is greater when contact with metal than with air. Therefore, holes in perforated shelf will result in non-uniform heat transfer, thus inhomogeneity in heat dependent reactions adversely effecting the direct quantitative analysis. It is preferable to keep the TLC plate down vertically, edges touching walls of the cup board. Hot plates with regulated range of temperature, i.e., 50-190°C ± 2°C are extensively being employed for heating the chromatogram. It has definite advantage — reaction can be followed visually, can be terminated as soon as optimal colour is developed and reagent's vapours will escape directly.

These reagents are most suited for glass-backed layers with inorganic binders. However suitability of plastic or aluminium-backed plates with organic binder shall have to be checked with each reagent-temperature combination. Such charring reagents produce coloured or fluorescent zones on heating (estimation of ethinylestradiol in oral contraceptive by converting it into fluorescent compound by treating with 10% v/v alcoholic sulphuric acid, and heating at 110°C for 5 min), prolonged heating is likely to char the whole plate. However, the intensity of the colour or fluorescence depends on duration of heating, temperature and solvent. Usually a temperature less than 120°C is employed. Aqueous or alcoholic (methanol or ethanol) solution of sulphuric acid (5-20%), 5% potassium dichromate solution in dilute sulphuric acid, 3% solution of cupric acetate in phosphoric acid or 2% ceric sulphate in 10% sulphuric acid are some of the classical charring reagents.

Note : Spraying of acid charring reagents is hazardous, should always be carried out in fume hood with extreme caution. Developed and dried TLC plate or sheet is placed on a sheet of filter paper, sprayed from a distance of about 15 cm with pressurized air. It is always preferable to spray the layer very thinly and evenly (with intermediate drying) than to saturate the layer with excessive spray reagent, as in the latter case, spots tend to diffuse.

A less hazardous charring reagent contains 10-20% ammonium sulphate mixed with the sorbent itself. The plate can be made in the laboratory by using aqueous solution of ammonium sulphate instead of water. Even precoated TLC plates containing ammonium sulphate are now commercially available. On heating at 150°C for 25-30 min, the salt decomposes to produce sulphuric acid in situ. Steroids (ethinylestradiol), triglycerides have been detected as fluorescent compounds when chromatographed on TLC plates containing ammonium sulphate.

While resorting to in situ pre- or postchromatographic derivatization followed by quantitative analysis, it is absolutely essential to ensure that reaction on the plate is complete or at least stoichiometric and reproducible. Dehydration reaction with sulphuric acid is often not stoichiometric and should be employed with care.

Both spraying (Fig. 7A & B) and dipping techniques are used for applying detection reagents. However, in addition to other reasons as enumerated below dipping followed by evaporation is essential both for precision and repeatability in ultimate quantitative analysis. The addition of reagents to mobile phase or stationary phase has been tried for detection and analysis such as ninhydrin can conveniently be added to mobile phase without altering the chromatographic profile for converting peptides or amino acids to coloured derivatives.

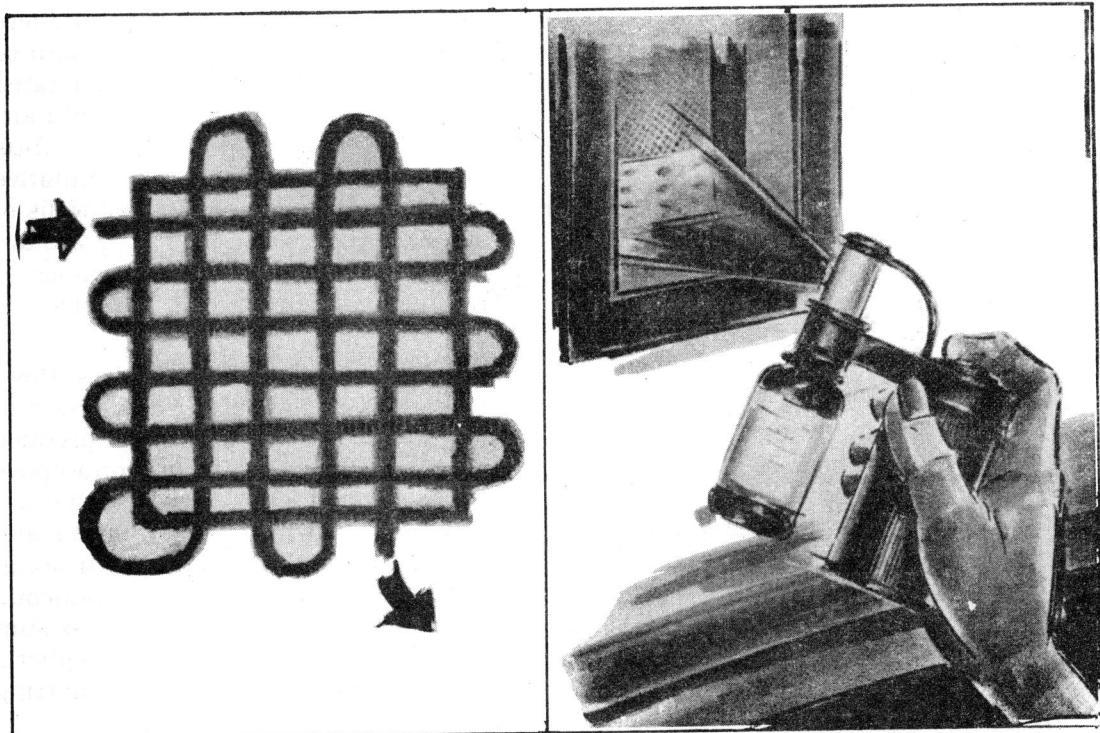

Fig. 7. A. Recommended spray scheme (meandering pattern). B. Spraying a TLC plate with the TLC-sprayer.

When the analyst has to resort to postchromatographic derivatization for detection or quantitative analysis, dipping technique for application of the reagent is preferred for following reasons :

- By using dipping techniques, the coating of the adsorbent layer with the reagent is more uniform.
- Distribution of the reagent is not influenced by viscosity of the reagent or drop size of spray mist.

- Detection limits are appreciably lower than in case of chromatogram sprayed as dipping transfers more reagent to the layer than spraying.
- Reproducibility of results is improved due to homogeneity of reagent application.
- Consumption of reagent is less.
- Reagent is less concentrated than used as spray.
- Contamination of the laboratory with the reagents particularly which are corrosive and hazardous/injurious to health such as sulphuric acid is less.
- Spray facilities such as fume cup board are not required.
- Results are more uniform, precise and reproducible.

Note : For derivatization, using dipping technique for application of the reagent, one is confronted with the risk that separated compounds may dissolve in the solvent present in the reagent or sorbent layer may get disturbed if the reagent is aqueous or polar solvents of the reagent may have elution effect on the fractions of the sample. It is therefore desirable that time of immersion in the reagent should be as short as possible but not more than five seconds to avoid dissolving of substances out of stationary phase. It is therefore more than necessary that due care should be taken in the choice of solvent for preparation of reagent solution. The solvent thus chosen should neither dissolve the separated substances nor their reaction products nor it should lead to tainting effect, otherwise ultimate analysis (quantitative) will be adversely effected. Further, after post-chromatographic derivatization if the plate is visually inspected, colour intensity of the zone must be more intense at the top surface of the layer than when it is viewed from back of the plate. If this is not the case, reagent must be made less polar to avoid development across the thickness of the layer.

Automated time controlled dipping apparatuses are now commercially available and are free from ripple effect which is usually observed with manual dipping technique.

Precautions

- Clean off back of the TLC plate which is wetted with the reagent before keeping it on hot plate, laboratory bench or scanning platform.
- Spraying of the reagent is not recommended particularly when ultimate aim is quantitative analysis as densitometric scanning of such plates results in irregular baseline.
- Protective glasses and laboratory gloves should always be worn during spraying.
- Propellant gases in ready to use spray guns contaminate the environment and well-ventilated fume cup board is essential to ensure effective removal of reagent clouds and toxic solvent vapours.
- Most of the chemical reactions proceed more rapidly at elevated temperature, heating at 100-110°C for 5-10 minutes is usually adequate to ensure complete reaction (with heating at higher temperature or for longer time, entire background of the plate tends to get darkened as binder present in the layer often char). In such case, silica gel H (without binder) may be suitable.
- For quantitative analysis after postderivatization, it is desired that heating if used should be uniform. Use of non-perforated stainless steel trays is recommended as support while drying in oven for uniform heat distribution.
- Although by spraying, uniform distribution of the reagent is difficult to achieve, however, in certain cases, it is unavoidable while using two or more reagents in sequence such as diazotization, followed by coupling with NED in case of sulphona-mides or conversion of thiamine hydrochloride (vitamin B_1) to a fluorescent derivative.

- Derivatization modifies or destroys the chemical structure of the compounds.
- Derivatization is more expensive and more complicated than detection with UV radiation but, in some cases, considerably more sensitive.
- On dipping there is a danger that the compounds will be dissolved out by the solvent used (consequence : change polarity) or that water in the dipping reagent may remove the layer (consequence : use reagent with organic solvents).
- Substances can diffuse during the dipping process.
- The detection reagent is distributed more uniformly in dipping than on spraying. Dipping reagents prove less of a hazard to personnel and the environment than sprays.
- On heating in a drying cabinet, a non-perforated metal tray should be used as a support to ensure uniform heat distribution.

Preparation of methanolic sulphuric acid : To 80-85 ml of ice-cold methanol while further cooling in freezing mixture, add cautiously and slowly 5-10 ml (as required) of sulphuric acid (already cooled in freezing mixture). Mix and make up the volume to 100 ml with ice-cooled methanol.

Almost every chemical reaction which can be performed in a test tube, can be carried out on a TLC layer.

Stabilization of developed spots/zones

After treatment with the reagent as part of chromatographic derivatization, coloured or fluorescent chromatographic zones are used for quantitative evaluation. It is therefore desirable that the colour or fluorescence thus produced should be stable at least for 30 minutes for carrying out various steps involved in quantitative analysis. There is no general procedure laid down to stabilize the coloured chromatographic zones except to store in atmosphere of nitrogen and protected from light till they are evaluated. However, fluorescent chromatographs can not only be stabilized but often intensified. For extensive details on stabilization and augmentation of fluorescence intensity, one may refer to compilation by Jork et al., 1990 & 1994.

For this, the developed chromatogram is dipped in viscous lipophilic (hydrophobic) solvents such as 10-20% solution of liquid paraffin (mineral oil) in n-hexane. The stabilization is due to exclusion of oxygen responsible for oxidative degradation of the substance. Mixture of chloroform–liquid paraffin–triethanolamine (60 + 10 + 10) has been employed in stabilizing and augmentation of fluorescence in case of thiamine hydrochloride (vitamin B_1) and ethinylestradiol (fluorescence is stable up to 24 h and usually two-fold augmentation is observed). Mixture of 33% liquid paraffin in cyclohexane has been employed for stabilizing and augmenting fluorescence in case of amiloride, aflatoxins, digitalis glycosides, fluphenazine, piroxicam, gentamycin, hydrophilic fluorescence intensifiers such as ethylene glycol, polyethylene glycol 400, 4000, triethylamine, triethanolamine triton X-100 are also employed.

Precautions

(a) For stabilizing the fluorescence, the plate may be immersed twice for 1 second each in the mixture of lipophilic solvent with brief intermediate drying.

(b) Quantitative evaluation should be resorted to at least 60 minutes after dipping as it takes longer time for fluorescent emission to stabilize.

Preparative thin layer chromatography

This technique is used when significant quantities of sample components are to be isolated and purified for subsequent analysis (IR, GC-MS, NMR).

- To achieve higher loading capacity, sample may be applied by streaking across the full width of the plate instead of spotting.
- Precoated plates of 20 cm height (20 × 20 cm) with a thickness up to 2000 μm are commercially available for preparative TLC. Preparative TLC plates (20 × 40 cm), 1000 μm thick have also been introduced by Whatman with product specification of PK5/4850940. (Whatman Chromatographic Folio — Publication No. 842 TLC PS).
- Laboratories having facilities for coating their own plates, can prepare plates of any height and thickness as required.
- Preparative plates having both preadsorbent and analytical layers are most suited for the purpose. Preadsorbent edge of the plate is dipped in the sample solution allowed to cover the preadsorbent area but before it reaches the interface with analytical area. The plate is taken out, dried and the process repeated. The plate is finally dried and subjected to development process as usual.
- Since sole purpose of preparative thin layer chromatography is to recover pure sample components, reversed-phase TLC plates give higher sample recovery, hence recommended particularly while dealing with valuable samples.
- After development, the plates should be dried in vacuum desiccator and never heated.
- No destructive detection technique should be used, most common technique being fluorescent quenching.
- Exposure to iodine vapours; the reaction with most of the compounds is reversible, but care should be taken to avoid oxidation.
- Spraying plates with water locates lipophilic and other water insoluble compounds.
- For eluting the detected zones, the entire plate should be sprayed to dampness with absolute alcohol, area marked and scrapped off with sharp blade, about 10% additional area than marked may preferably be scrapped to compensate for 3-dimensional development of the band in the layer.
- Minimum volume of the solvent should be used for eluting the components from scrapped material, usually mobile phase is recommended for the purpose. Volume of solvent required can be calculated as follows :

  Volume of solvent required = Volume of scrapped material × 10 × (1 − Rf)

  For eluting 0.5 ml of scrapped material of sample with Rf value of 0.2, we require 0.4 ml of the solvent.

  Volume of solvent required = 0.5 × 10 × (1 − 0.2) = 0.4 ml.
- Scrapped material and solvent is homogenised in vortex mixture to ensure complete elution, centrifuged, supernatant collected for evaporation.
- Solvent mixtures containing 20-30% methanol are preferred.

One may also encounter the following problems in preparative chromatography :

1. Sample may be lost through irreversible adsorption — can be minimised by using reversed-phase chromatography.
2. Contamination from other sources.
   (a) Solvent : Use chromatographic grade solvent.
   (b) TLC plates : Prewash the plate before use and always store in vacuum desiccator.

Reversed-phase TLC/HPTLC

Most separation by TLC is performed with unmodified silica gel precoated layers. However due to complexity of certain separation problems and in response to the increasing demands and expectation of chromatographers to design mobile phases for HPLC without involving risk to costly columns, new layers with chemically modified silica gel have been introduced. Selectivity of adsorbent is continuously being increased by chemical modification of the layers, some of the most common modifications are amino, cyano, diol and silanization (commonly represented as RP_2, RP_8 and RP_{18}). The use of silanized (reversed-phase) plates provide quick and inexpensive previewed separation traits prior to HPLC (an estimated 80-90% of HPLC analysis is performed using reversed-phase columns). While using reversed-phase layers, it is relatively easier to find a good mobile phase as there are only a few volatile water miscible solvents available and most of them are generally found suitable such as methanol, acetonitrile, dioxane. It is increasingly being experienced that different components of a formulation which could not be resolved using normal-phase TLC could easily be resolved by reversed phase TLC often resulting in partial or complete reversal of retention order (Figs. 12 and 13). Substances migrate in a general order of decreasing polarity (the most polar solute moves the fastest) and mobile phase strength increases with decreasing polarity (acetonitrile is a stronger solvent than water). On the other hand, wide variety of mobile phases available for use in normal-phase silica gel TLC increases separation potential. HPTLC silica gel 60 with a mean particle size of 6 nm and mean pore size of 60 Å is used for RP precoated plates. Octadecyl chains are chemically bounded to the silanol groups (Fig. 2) on the surface of silica gel. These layers are designed to correlate to C_{18} bounded HPLC reversed-phase columns (usually 10-12% carbon loading). Chemically bound octadecyl chains are responsible for the reversed-phase character of the layer, remaining silanol groups which are not converted determine the hydrophilic properties of the sorbent, thus degree of wettability. Lower the modification, lesser the interaction between solute and sorbent, hence higher Rf value.

Note : Difference between Rf values with mobile phase of similar eluotropic strength are much lower than silica gel. Therefore in identity testing by RPTLC, use of more than one mobile phase does not elicit much additional information.

Sample preparation

The samples spotted onto a RPHPTLC plate shall meet the same requirements as for normal-phase silica gel HPTLC. The samples that require extraction and clean-up prior to cellulose or silica gel TLC can sometime be applied directly to RP plates, such as analysis of dyes in suspension and syrups and food products, the sample need only be diluted with methanol prior to RPTLC.

As RPTLC plates have high capacity and can accept large quantity of samples, clean-up of the sample or its concentration is often not necessary. Because of high capacity, less concentrated sample solution can be employed, thus reducing the need for plates with preadsorbent or preconcentration layers.

Standards and samples should be dissolved in most polar solvent to avoid band spreading. By using weak solvent, purification of the complex samples is also achieved as highly non-polar impurities get eliminated being insoluble in weak solvents (selective solvation). Taking into consideration the stability of the compounds, wettability limitations, sample solutions should be prepared in predominantly organic solvent than in water. Methanol which is quickly evaporated and usually wets the layers adequately is suitable for substances capable of hydrogen bonding. For less polar compounds, methylene chloride and acetone are the suitable solvents.

Mobile phase selection

The greatest advantage of RPTLC is the simplicity of mobile phase. This is usually a two component mixture of water and a polar organic solvent miscible with water such as methanol, acetonitrile, acetone, dioxane. By adjusting the proportions of the components of the mobile phase, separation can be tuned. As a rule, more non-polar the sample, higher the proportion of organic component of the mobile phase. As polarity of the mobile phase increases, so does the contents of water in the mobile phase. While using water-alcohol mixtures as mobile phase, resolution may be improved by changing the alcohol to one of higher or lower chain lengths with constant concentration or by altering the alcohol–water ratio such as methanol ↔ ethanol ↔ propanol.

To start with chromatographic work with RPTLC, mixture of ethanol–water (80 : 20 v/v) is the most useful starting mobile phase. Selectivity may be improved by altering the ratio with water. Addition of 1-20% of tetrahydrofuran or dimethylformamide can prove useful in difficult separation problems. Mixtures of water with polar solvents often offer wettability problem. Separation of organic acid is facilitated by addition of weak acid such as formic acid or acetic acid to the mobile phase to give a pH value below the pH of the acid solutes.

Solvent mixtures containing more than 40% water may damage binding properties of the layer in addition to wettability problem, bad spot shape and irregular solvent front. This can be overcome by adding ion-pair salts or sodium chloride (0.1 to 0.5 M) instead of water. The addition of salt usually does not affect the separation, rather increases the migration rate of the mobile phase. Addition of 0.5 M sodium chloride to acetonitrile-water mixture containing less than 25% of water, usually demixing of phase is observed, then ammonium acetate (0.5 M) may be employed instead of sodium chloride.

- RP plates normally do not require activation.
- Adjustment of water content is not critical as with silica gel because virtually all accessible silanol groups are de-activated by chemical bonding with hydrocarbons.
- Solvent demixing is less of a problem.
- Independent of humidity.
- Non-chlorinated solvents.
- Higher the percentage of carbon loading of the layer, more the developing time, usually carbon loading of about 12% gives good results.
- Rate of development decreases with increasing water contents of mobile phase.
- Chemically bonded RP layers offer advantage over otherwise impregnated layers (with paraffin oil or silicone oil) of non-contamination of solute with impregnating liquid.

Note :

1. While using neutral solvents (methanol/water), if the coated surface is damaged, use of 0.5 M sodium chloride will prevent the damage to some extent.

2. Bonded layers can be washed with methanol, acetone, methylene chloride and re-used several times with no apparent change in chromatographic separation profile. Washing is usually continued till previously chromatographed spots are undetected under UV.

Common TLC Equipments and Accessories

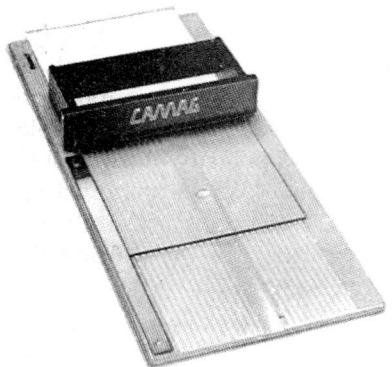

Fig. 1. Manual TLC plate coater.

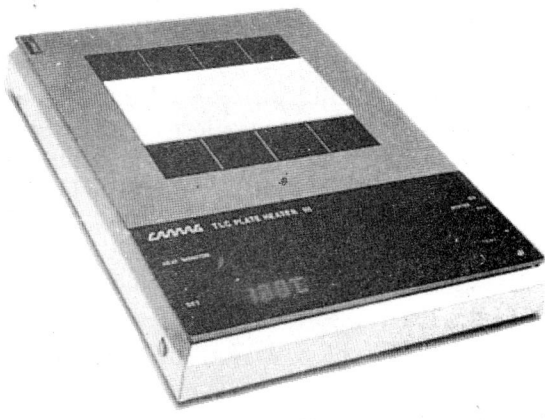

Fig. 4. TLC plate heater, selectable **temperature** range between 25° and 200°C, **programmable.**

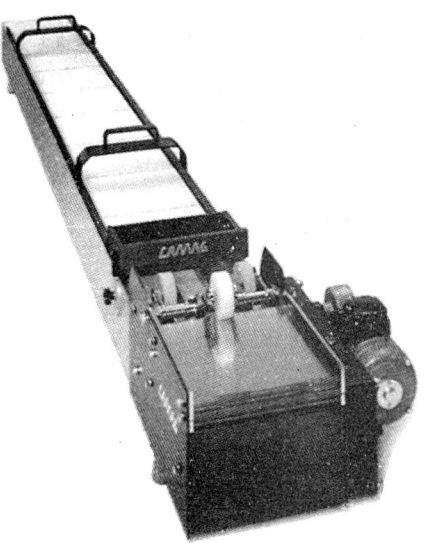

Fig. 2. Automatic TLC plate coater.

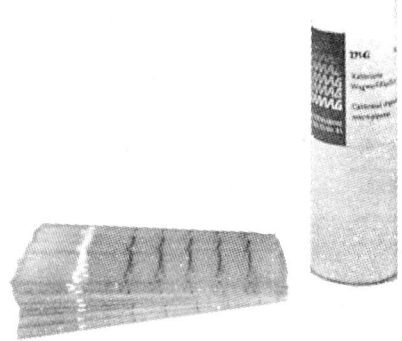

Fig. 5. Graduated glass capillaries (5 μl), suitable for qualitative analysis.

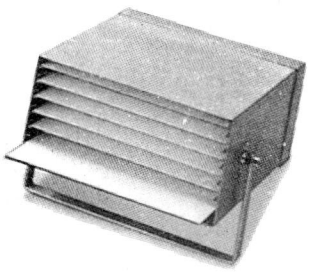

Fig. 3. TLC plate box, suitable to hold 20 × 20 cm plates for drying or re-activation of plates.

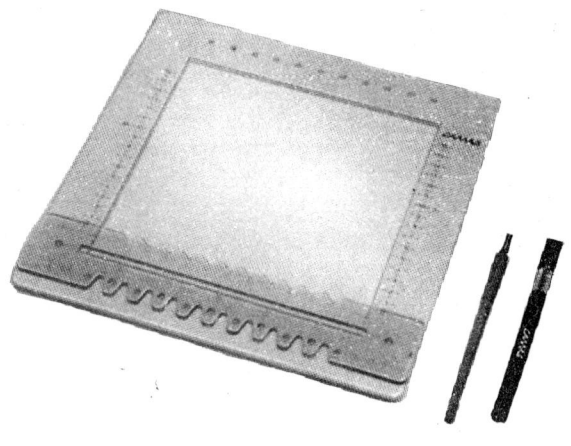

Fig. 6. Multipurpose spotting guide.

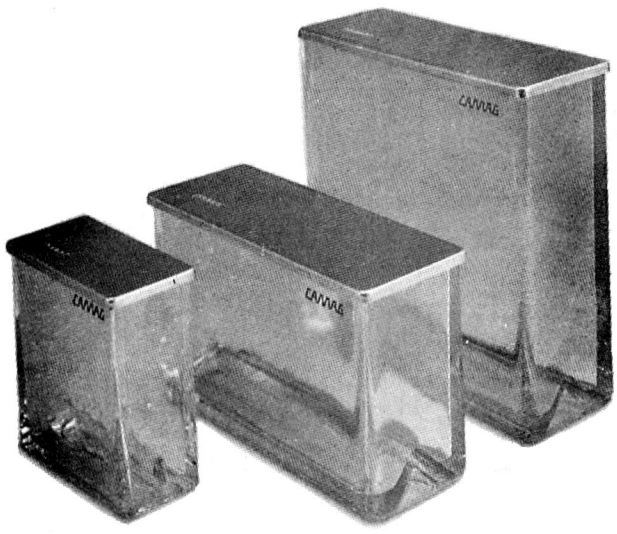

Fig. 7. Twin-trough chambers with lids.

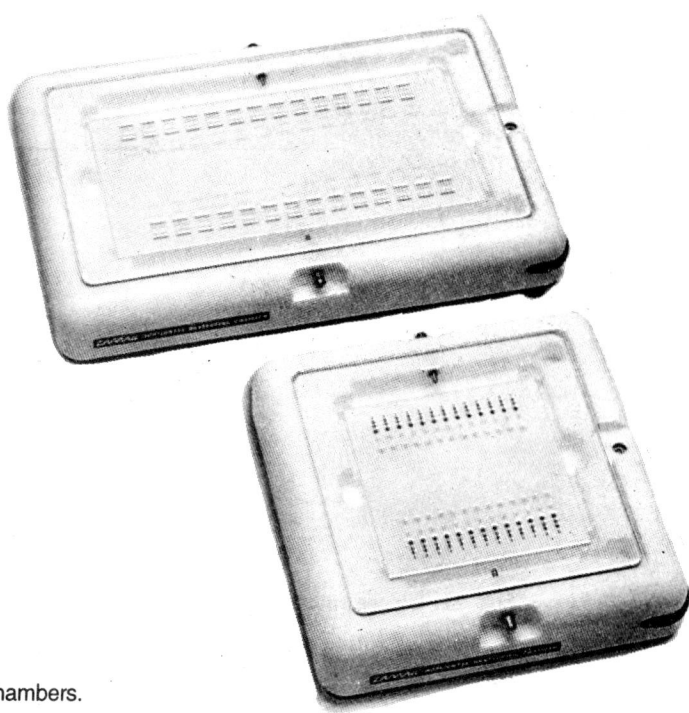

Fig. 8. Horizontal developing chambers.

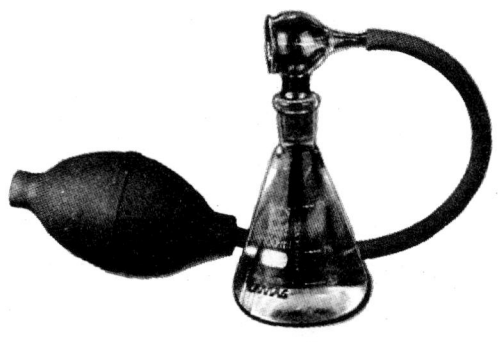

Fig. 9. All-glass sprayer (atomizer).

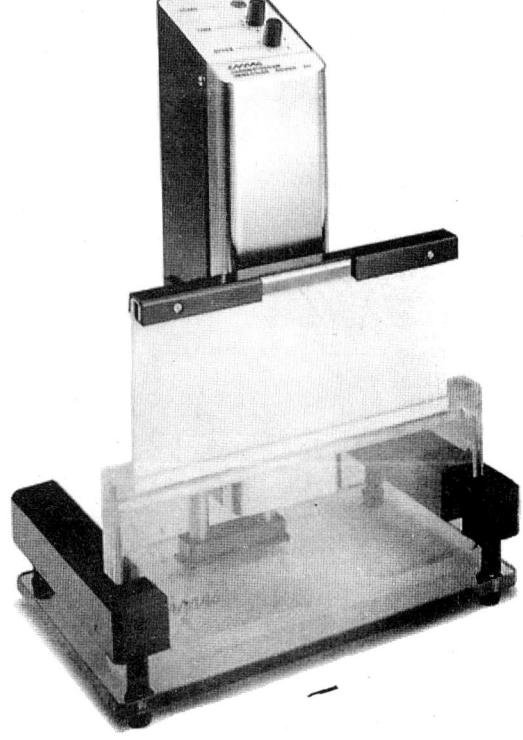

Fig. 11. Immersion device with selectable immersion speed and time.

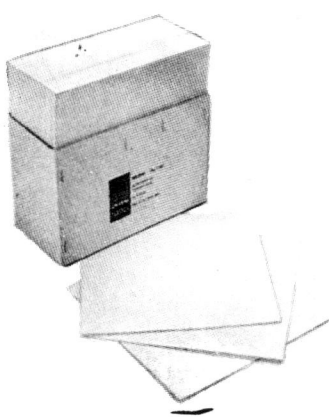

Fig. 10. Saturation pads made of thick filter paper for lining inner wall of the developing chamber.

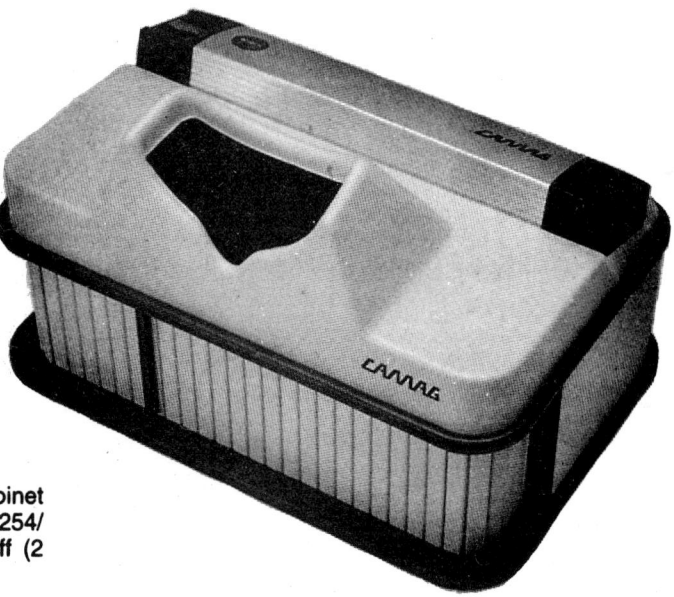

Fig. 12. UV-viewing cabinet with dual wavelength (254/ 366 nm) and auto-cutoff (2 min) device.

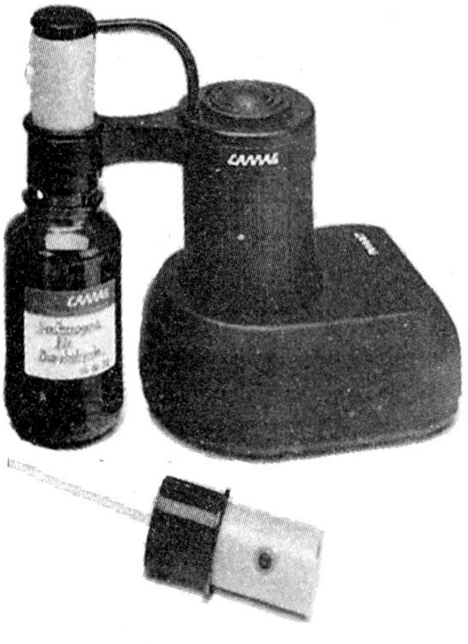

Fig. 13. TLC sprayer, cordless, suitable for spraying solutions of normal and high viscosity.

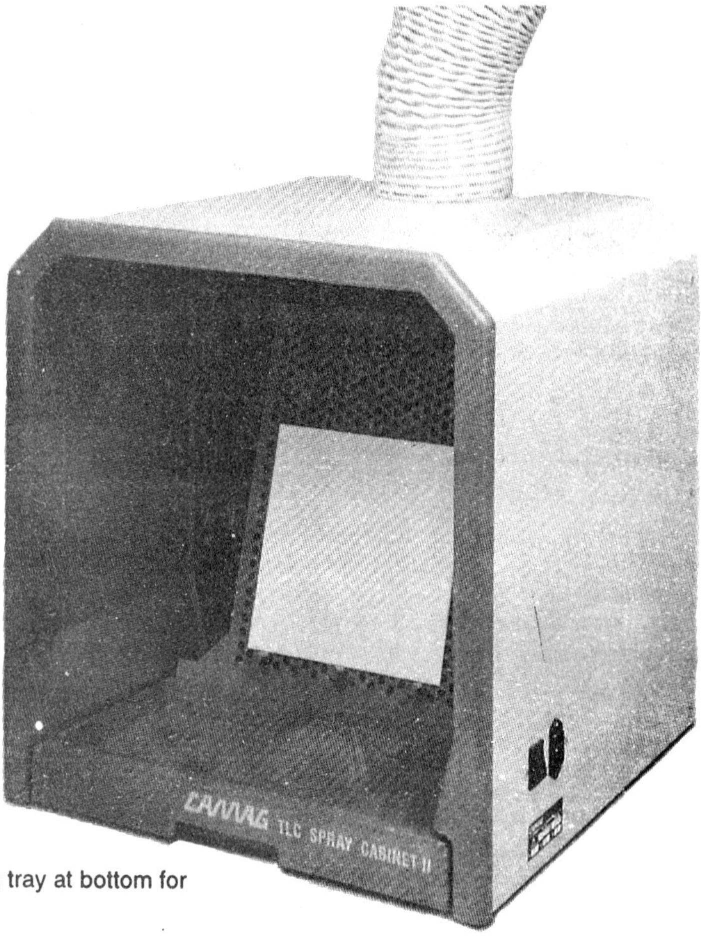

Fig. 14. TLC spray cabinet with built-in tray at bottom for easy cleaning.

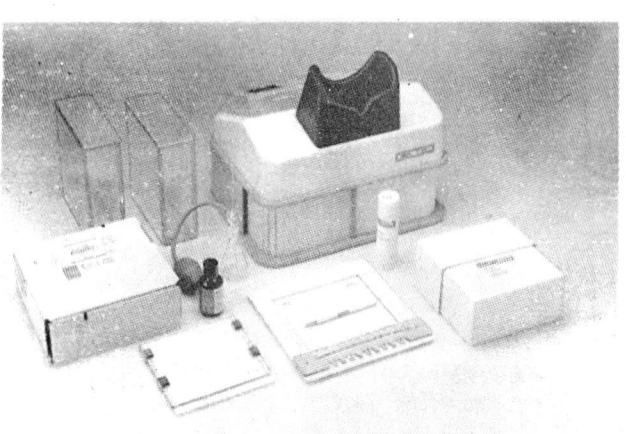

Fig. 15. TLC basic kit consisting of multipurpose spotting guide; micro-capillaries (5 μl); flat bottom and twin-trough chamber; all-glass reagent sprayer; UV-viewing cabinet filled with short (254 nm) and long (365 nm) wavelength lamps; pre-coated TLC plates and test dye mixture.

Figs. 1 to 15 courtesy Camag, Switzerland, through Anchrom Enterprises (I) Pvt. Ltd., Mumbai, India.

Common Detection and Visualization Reagents

"Best of separation techniques are of no avail if the results of separation cannot be detected."

All the drugs of interest are not detectable in visible range. They are located by their response to UV light and their reaction with various sequence of spray reagents. TLC plates containing a fluorescent indicator are preferably used so that the first step to locate the substance shall be to examine the plate under short (254 nm) and long (365 nm) ultraviolet light to detect both absorbing and fluorescent spots.

Although, colour obtained with different spray reagents is a good guide, but factors such as quantity of the drug spotted, pH and the amount of spray reagent will alter the hue and intensity of colour obtained.

Colour reactions are more or less clearly defined reactions of substances with suitable reagent. Substance-specific reactions are usually not available and many compounds with aromatic structure give positive Marquis' reaction. Aldehydes react with electron-rich compounds in acidic medium to yield coloured compounds. Colour reactions are more useful if it is known that a particular functional group is present in the molecule; this only increases the specificity of evidence, but does not allow the direct identification. Chromatographic separation before detection is an important tool for increasing the specificity towards the reagent.

It is often possible to increase the specificity and selectivity of detection by carrying out sequence of reactions on the plate after chromatographic development. This technique is called "reagent sequences".

Reagents

1. Hydrochloric acid vapours : Generated by keeping 10 ml of fuming HCl in one trough of twin-trough chamber (for hydrolysis).
2. (a) 10% w/v solution of sodium nitrite in water.
   (b) Dilute hydrochloric acid (10%) (for diazotization).
3. 5% solution of ammonium sulphamate (for destruction of excess nitrite).
4. 0.5% solution of n-naphthyl–ethylene diamine (NED) in methanol (coupling for formation of azo-dye).

The dried chromatogram is exposed to HCl vapors (reagent 1) for few seconds and then heated at 110°C for 5 min to remove excess of HCl vapours. After cooling, the plate is successively sprayed with reagents 2a and 2b, dried briefly and then sprayed with reagent 3, dried and finally sprayed with reagent 4. Red azo-dye on a light background is produced.

Reaction sequence for detection of hydrochlorothiazide on TLC plate

MOST COMMONLY USED DETECTION REAGENTS

A. Basic nitrogenous drug substances

1. Ninhydrin spray : Spray the plate with the reagent and heat at 100°C for 5 min. Violet to pink spots for primary amines and yellow for secondary amines.
2. FPN reagent : This reagent is commonly used to over-spray a plate which has previously been sprayed with ninhydrin.
3. Dragendorff's reagent : Yellow, orange, red-orange or brown-orange spots are often observed; suitable for alkaloids.
4. Acidified iodoplatinate solution : Violet, blue-violet, grey-violet or brown-violet spots observed with quaternary ammonium compounds.
5. Marquis reagent : Violet spots observed; suitable for opium alkaloids.
6. Acidified potassium permanganate solution : Yellow-brown spots against violet background obtained.

B. Acidic drug substances

1. Van Urk reagent : After spraying, heat the plate at 100°C for 5 min. Yellow spots (sulphonamides) and blue spots (ergot alkaloids) obtained.
2. Ferric (iron) chloride solution : Blue or violet spots are obtained with phenolic substances.
3. Acidified potassium permanganate solution, suitable for phenolic substances.
4. Mercuric nitrate solution suitable for barbiturates.

C. Neutral drug substances

1. Furfuraldehyde reagent.
2. Acidified iodoplatinate solution.
3. Acidified potassium permanganate solution.

1. Acidified iodoplatinate reagent

Preparation : Dissolve 0.25 g of platinic chloride and 5 g of potassium iodide in 90 ml of water, add 5 ml of hydrochloric acid and make up the volume to 100 ml with water.

The reagent is used for the detection of the following drug substances :

Amiloride HCl, amodiaquine, antazoline, atropine, benzhexol, berberine, betaine, bisacodyl, bromhexine, brucine, buclizine, caffeine, carbinoxamine, cetylpyridinium chloride, chlordiazepoxide, chlorhexidine, chloroquine, chlorpheniramine, chlorpromazine, cinnarizine, clidinium bromide, clonidine, codeine, cyclizine, cyproheptadine, dextromethorphan, dextropropoxyphene, diazepam, diloxanide furoate, dimethindene, diphenhydramine hydrochloride, diphenoxylate hydrochloride, diphenylpyraline hydrochloride, dipyridamole, dipyrone, domiphen bromide, emetine hydrochloride, ephedrine hydrochloride, ethylmorphine, fenfluramine, glibenclamide, haloperidol, chlorquinol (8-OH quinoline), hydralazine hydrochloride, hydroxyzine hydrochloride, hyoscine hydrobromide, hyoscyamine sulphate, imipramine HCl, isoniazid lignocaine HCl, lorazepam, meclozine HCl, mepyramine, metoclopramide HCl, morphine sulphate, naphazoline, nitrazepam, nortriptyline, noscapine, orphenadrine HCl, papaverine, phenazone, pheniramine maleate, phenylpropanolamine, pilocarpine, pipenzolate bromide, promethazine, propranolol, pyrantel, pyrimethamine, selegiline, thiacetazone, thiabendazole, thiamine, trifluoperazine, xylometazoline.

2. Alizarin reagent

Preparation : 0.25% w/v solution of alizarin in methanol. The solution can be kept for several days at room temperature. It yields coloured complexes with metals of various categories such as Cu^+, Ag^+, Ca^{++}, Sr^{++}, Ba^{++}, Al^{+++}.

The developed chromatogram is dried in warm air for 10 min and sprayed evenly with the solution. While the plate is still moist, it is exposed to ammonia vapours. In few minutes, red-violet spots appear against violet background. To improve the contrast, dip the plate in boric acid solution (1% in 90% methanol), background turns yellow. 1% acetic acid in ether may be used instead of boric acid solution.

Note :
1. Instead of dipping in boric acid or acetic acid solution, heat the plate to 100°C for 3-5 min in fume cupboard to evaporate ammonia and to turn the background yellow. This treatment increases the sensitivity of detection of some cations such as Sr^{++}, Ba^{++}.
2. The coloured spots so obtained tend to fade away after some time. The reagent is suitable for silica gel or cellulose layers.

3. Aluminium chloride reagent

1% w/v solution of aluminium chloride hexahydrate in methanol. The solution can be stored for a long period in the refrigerator. The reagent forms fluorescent complexes with flavonoids such as rutin, quercetin, hespiridine. The developed chromatogram, when sprayed or dipped in the reagent and air-dried, reveals yellow fluorescent spots when examined under long-wave UV (365 nm). Heating at 85-90°C for few minutes increases the sensitivity as compared to air-drying. The reagent is suitable for silica gel, kieselguhr, polyamide, RP layers, modified (CN, NH_2) and cellulose layers.

For detection of triglycerides, cholesterol, mycotoxins, spraying with stronger solution is necessary.

4. 4-aminoantipyrine–potassium ferricyanide reagent (Emerson reagent)

Solution 1 : 1% w/v solution of 4-aminoantipyrine in 80% methanol.

Solution 2 : 40% w/v solution of potassium ferricyanide in 50% methanol.

The solutions can be stored in refrigerator for 7 days.

4-aminoantipyrine forms with amines coloured diimine derivative due to oxidative action of iron (III) ions.

After development, the chromatogram is freed from mobile phase, it is sprayed with solution 1, dried in warm air for 5 min, and then sprayed with solution 2. After drying, the plate is placed in chamber with ammonia vapours for decolourizing the background (ensure that layer does not come in contact with liquid).

Red-orange coloured zones are produced against pale-yellow background.

The reagent can be employed on silica gel, kieselguhr, aluminium oxide, polyamide, RP and NH_2 layers.

The reagent can be used for detection of eugenol, thymol, phenylephrine, amoxycillin, salbutamol, piroxicam, doxycycline, triamcinolone, niclosamide and various other drug substances containing phenolic (OH) functional group.

5. 4-aminobenzoic acid reagent

Preparation : 0.5 g of p-aminobenzoic acid (PABA) is dissolved in 9 ml of glacial acetic acid, add 10 ml of water, 1 ml of phosphoric acid (total volume 20 ml).

The reagent may be stored for 7 days in the dark at room temperature. Just before use, dilute 10 ml of the above solution to 25 ml of acetone and use as spray solution. After development, the chromatogram is freed from mobile phase, and sprayed with the spray solution till the plate is completely moistened. Heat the plate at 120°C for 10-15 min, coloured spots which fluoresce under long wavelength UV light (365 nm) are obtained. This reagent can be employed on silica gel and cellulose layers.

The reagent is used for detection of carbohydrates (monosaccharides, disaccharides such as lactose, fructose, glucose). Sugars react with the reagent to form Schiff's base.

6. Ammonia vapour reagent

Ammonia solution : 25%

May be stored in cool place over extended period of time.

After development, the chromatogram is freed from mobile phase and exposed to ammonia vapours for 15 min in twin-trough chamber. Examine under long wavelength UV light (365 nm). Yellow, green or blue fluorescent spots are observed against dark background.

The reagent can be employed on silica gel, kieselguhr, polyamide, RP and cellulose layers.

The reagent is used for detection of opium alkaloids (morphine, heroin, ethyl-morphine), flavonoids, flavonoid glycosides, sennosides (A and B), antibiotics (penicillins, rifamycin, tetracyclines), anthracene derivatives, mycotoxins.

7. Ammonium monovanadate–sulphuric acid reagent (Mandelin's reagent)

Spray solution :

la : Saturated solution of ammonium monovanadate in concentrated sulphuric acid.

lb : Dissolve 1.2 g of ammonium vanadate in 95 ml water and carefully add 5 ml of conc. sulphuric acid. Yellow coloured vanadyl (V) ion is converted to blue vanadyl (IV) ion by reaction with reducing agent.

After development, remove the mobile phase and then spray with the reagent (1a or 1b) until the layer is transparent. Then heat at 105°C for 5 min, cool and again spray lightly. The reagent is suitable for silica gel, kieselguhr and cellulose layers. It is used for detection of carbohydrates, glycols (glycerin, diethylene glycol, propylene glycols, ethylene glycol), reducing carboxylic acids (ascorbic acid), steroids, antioxidants, phenols, aromatic amino compounds. The reagent 1a is specific for β-blockers (acebutalol, propranolol, atenolol, pindolol, alprenolol, dihydralazine).

8. Aniline–diphenylamine–phosphoric acid reagent

Spray solution : Transfer 1 ml of aniline to 75 ml of methanol, add 1 g of di-phenylamine and after addition of 10 ml of phosphoric acid dilute to 100 ml with methanol.

The developed chromatogram is freed from mobile phase and spray evenly with the solution. The plate is heated at 90-110°C for 15-20 min and observe the development of coloured spots while the plate is being dried (temperature and duration of heating affect colour development).

The reagent is suitable for silica gel, kieselguhr and modified (NH_2, CN) layers. The reagent is commonly used for detection of sugars (ketohexoses, pentoses), glucoronic acid and galactoronic acid.

9. Anisaldehyde–sulphuric acid reagent

Spray solution : Add carefully 8 ml of conc. sulphuric acid to 0.5 ml of anisaldehyde (ice-cooled), while keeping in ice-bath during addition add 85 ml of methanol and 10 ml of glacial acetic acid. Use of freezing mixture is preferred than ice-bath.

After development, remove the mobile phase with stream of warm air and then spray homogeneously with the spray solution until the layer is transparent. Then heat the plate to 100-150°C for 5-10 min (background tends to acquire reddish colourisation if heating is carried out too long; can be decolorised by treating with water). Coloured fluorescent spots are observed when examined under long wavelength UV light (365 nm). It is a universal reagent for natural products.

The reagent is suitable for silica gel, kieselguhr and RP layers. It can be used for detection of antioxidants, steroids, prostaglandins, carbohydrates, cardiac· glycosides, antibiotics (macrolides and tetracyclines), mycotoxins, essential oil components (menthol, thymol, carophylline) and other common drug substances such as paracetamol, analgin, chlordiazepoxide, amoxycillin, isoniazid, promethazine, phenothiazines, metoclopramide, benzocaine, chlorthalidone.

10. Antimony (III) chloride reagent (Carr–Price reagent)

Spray solution : 10% w/v solution of antimony chloride in carbon tetrachloride (solution should be freshly prepared).

After development, remove mobile phase and spray evenly with spray solution and heat at 110-120°C for 5-10 min. Coloured fluorescent spots are observed when examined under long wavelength UV light (365 nm). The reagent is suitable for silica gel, kieselguhr and aluminium oxide layers.

The reagent is specifically used for estimation of vitamin D_2, D_3 and A and for carotenoids, terpenes, triterpenes, sterols, steroids (hormones and alkaloids), cholic acid, cardiac glycosides, flavonoids.

11. 2,2'-bipyridine–iron (III) chloride reagent (Emmerie–Engel reagent)

Spray solution :

(a) 0.2% w/v solution of ferric chloride in methanol.

(b) 0.5% w/v solution of 2,2'-bipyridine (α-α'-dipyridyl) in methanol.

Mix equal quantities of solution (a) and (b) immediately before use.

Remove the mobile phase with the aid of warm air. Spray with the solution and then dry with cold air. Reddish-brown spots are visible against colourless background. The spots often appear after 20-30 min.

· The reagent is suitable for silica gel and cellulose layer.

The reagent is used for detection of reducing agents such as ascorbic acid. Iron (II) produced as result of reduction of iron (III) reacts with dipyridyl to give the colour. Vitamin E, salbutamol, terbutaline, phenols and antioxidants can be detected with this reagent.

12. Blue tetrazolium reagent

Spray solution :

(a) 0.5% w/v solution of tetrazolium blue in methanol.

(b) Dissolve 20 g of sodium hydroxide in 50 ml of water and dilute to 100 ml with methanol.

Just before use, mix equal volumes of solution (a) and (b). 20 ml of this solution is mixed with 40 ml of methanol to be used as spray solution.

Both solutions (a) and (b) can be separately stored for extended period in refrigerator. The chromatogram is evenly sprayed. Violet coloured spots are immediately visible against light background at room temperature (gentle heating may sometime be required).

The reagent is suitable for silica gel, aluminium oxide, polyamide and cellulose layers.

The reagent may be used for detection of corticosteroids (dexamethasone, beta-methasone, cortisone, prednisolone, hydrocortisone), isosorbide, spironolactone, beclomethasone, clobetasol and pyraquantel.

13. Bratton–Marshall reagent

Spray solutions :

1. (a) 5% solution of sodium nitrite in water.

   (b) Mix 15 ml of conc. hydrochloric acid with 85 ml methanol.

   Mix 20 ml of solution (1a) with (1b) just before spraying.

2. 0.5% solution of N-(1-naphthyl), ethylene diamine dihydrochloride in methanol.

3. 5% solution of ammonium sulphamate.

For its use, refer to page 34 under reaction sequence. The reagent is suitable for silica gel, cellulose and RP layers.

The reagent is used for detection of substances having primary aromatic amines (sulphonamides). Other common substances detected are benzocaine, bromhexine, captopril, metoclopramide, folic acid, nimuselide, phenylbutazone, diazepam.

14. Bromocresol purple or bromocresol green reagent

Spray solution : 0.1% solution of bromocresol purple or green in methanol, add few drops of 10% ammonia till colour changes.

After the mobile phase is removed with the stream of warm air, the chromatogram is evenly sprayed with the solution and then heated to 100°C for few minutes. Lemon-yellow spots appear against blue-black background in case of organic acids, whereas halide ions yield yellow spots. The reagent is suitable for silica gel, kieselguhr, and cellulose layers. The reagent may be used for detection of acids (lactic acid, tartaric acid, malic acid, succinic acid, fumaric acid, citric acid and salicylic acid) and other acidic drug substances such as ketotifen, ibuprofen, oxyphenbutazone, diclofenac, ticlopidine, fenfluramine, ketoconazole, albendazole, loperamide, amodiaquine, hydroxyzine, prazosine, orphenadrine.

Note : Fading of developed colours can be delayed by covering the chromatogram with a glass plate.

15. N-bromosuccinimide reagent

Spray solution : 0.5% w/v solution of n-bromosuccinimide in acetone or n-butanol. The reagent can be stored in refrigerator for a week.

After the chromatogram is freed from mobile phase, it is sprayed with the solution; yellow to brown coloured spots are observed which emit pale-blue fluorescence on dark background when examined under long wavelength UV light (365 nm).

The reagent is suitable for silica gel, kieselguhr and cellulose layers. It can be used for detection of amino acids, flavonoids (rutin, quercetin, hespiridine), hydroxyquinoline derivatives, amoxycillin, amodiaquine.

16. p-chloranil reagent

Spray solution : 0.2% solution of tetrachloro-p-benzoquinone in toluene or dioxane or ethylacetate or acetonitrile.

The reagent is stable for 7 days when stored in refrigerator.

Remove the mobile phase with the help of stream of warm air and then spray evenly with the solution. The plate may be heated (105-110°C for 2 min) to accelerate the reaction as well as to enhance the colour intensity. The reagent is suitable for silica gel, RP-8, RP-18, and modified (NH_2, CN, Diol) layers. The reagent is used for detection of aromatic amines (sulphonamides), alkaloids (ephedrine, piperazine, emetine, reserpine, berberine, morphine, papaverine) local anaesthetics (procaine, lidocaine), phenothiazine derivatives (promethazine, promazine), benzodiazepines (chlordiazepoxide, diazepam), antibiotics (ampicillin, amoxycillin, cloxacillin, dicloxacillin), diuretics (acetazolamide, furosemide), antidiabetics (tolubutamide, gliclazide), cardiac drugs (metoprolol, propranolol).

17. Copper (II) nitrate reagent

Spray solution : Dilute 1 ml of saturated aqueous solution of copper (II) nitrate to 100 ml with methanol, add 0.2 ml of 10% nitric acid. The reagent is very stable.

The coloured spots obtained with ninhydrin in case of amino acids tend to fade rapidly. The stability of the colour is enhanced by forming complex with metal ions. Common metal ions used for complex formation are Co^{++}, Cu^{++}, Cd^{++}, Zn^{++}. After the chromatogram is sprayed with ninhydrin, it is sprayed with copper nitrate solution and then exposed to ammonia vapours placed in twin-trough chamber. Amino acids yield reddish spots against highly brown background. These spots are quite stable for considerable time. The reagent is used to stabilize amino acids–ninhydrin spots.

18. 2,6-dibromoquinone-4-chloroimide reagent (Gibbs' reagent)

Spray solution : Dissolve 0.5 g of 2,6-dibromoquinone-4-chloroimide (DBQC) in 100 ml of methanol. The solution is likely to decompose explosively; so small quantity should be stored in refrigerator.

The chromatogram is dried by cold air and then heated to 110°C, cooled and sprayed with DBQC solution and heated to 110°C for 2 min, cooled and exposed to ammonia (25%) vapours.

The reagent is suitable for silica gel, polyamide, and cellulose layers.

The reagent can be used for detection of phenols, primary, secondary and tertiary aromatic amines which are not substituted in the p-position. Common drug substances which can be detected are salicylamide, piperazine, amoxycillin, oxyphenbutazone, salbutamol, primaquine, resorcinol, thymol, rifampicin, cloxacillin, 8-OH-quinolines, piroxicam, cimetidine, carbamezepine, cumarins, isoxsuperine, thiamine, nylidrin, pyridoxine, stanozalol, barbiturates.

19. 2,6-dichlorophenol indophenol reagent (Tillman's reagent)

Spray solution : 0.1% solution of 2,6-dichlorophenol indophenol in methanol.

The reagent may be stored in refrigerator in air-tight container for several months.

The chromatogram is air-dried (to remove mobile phase) and then sprayed with the solution followed by heating at 100°C for 5 min. Acids normally yield red-orange spots whereas reducing agents (ascorbic acid) produce colourless spots on blue-violet background. The reagent is suitable for silica gel, kieselguhr, polyamide and cellulose layers. The reagent can be used for detection of organic acids (tartaric acid, malic acid, lactic acid, succinic acid, fumaric acid) and reducing agents (ascorbic acid).

20. 2,6-dichloroquinone-4-chloroimide reagent

For its preparation and application refer to 2,6-dibromoquinone-4-chloroimide reagent (Gibbs' reagent).

21. 4-(dimethylaminobenzaldehyde)-acid reagent

4-(dimethylaminobenzaldehyde)-PDAB is the main component in all these reagents, the difference being in the type and concentration of mineral acid used in the preparation. Two most commonly used reagents are as per their inventors :

(a) Ehrlich's reagent

(b) Van Urk's reagent

Ehrlich's reagent uses hydrochloric acid, whereas Urk's reagent contains sulphuric acid.

Ehrlich's reagent is usually more sensitive for in-situ evaluation, however the plate background is yellow in colour whereas in the case or Urk's reagent it is white or very light grey and does not discolour on standing. However, Ehrlich's reagent is more commonly employed for TLC identification.

Ehrlich's reagent

Spray solution : 1% w/v solution of PDAB in concentrated hydrochloric acid–methanol (1 : 1). The reagent is quite stable.

After drying with the aid of warm air, spray the chromatogram with the solution till the layer is transparent. Heat the plate at 50°C for 10-15 minutes, coloured spots appear against light yellow background.

The reagent is suitable for silica gel, aluminium oxide, kieselguhr, cellulose, RP-8, RP-18, impregnated ($AgNO_3$) and chiral layers.

The reagent is used for detection of drug substances such as sulphonamides, bromhexine, paracetamol, chlordiazepoxide, benzocaine, thiacetazone, isoniazid, oxyphenbutazone, amoxycillin, ergot alkaloids, phenothiazines, indomethazine, barbiturates, terbutaline, chlorthalidone, metoclopramide.

Van Urk's reagent

Spray solution : Dissolve 50 mg of PDAB in methanol–sulphuric acid (98%)— (90 : 10).

The solution is sprayed till the chromatogram is transparent. Heat the plate at 105-110°C for 10 min; coloured spots against colourless background are obtained. The reagent is suitable for silica gel, aluminium oxide, kieselguhr layers. The reagent is used for detection of ergot and tropane alkaloids, lysergic acid derivatives, sulphonamides and other compounds containing primary aromatic group.

22. 4-(dimethylamino)-benzaldehyde–acetylacetone reagent (Morgan–Elson reagent)

Spray solution : Dissolve 1 g of 4-dimethylaminobenzaldehyde in 30 ml of methanol and 30 ml of conc. hydrochloric acid (fuming).

To be prepared just before use.

Dried chromatogram is sprayed with the reagent and then heated at 105°C for 5 min, cool and again spray with the reagent and again heat at 90°C for 5 min. Red to brown spots are produced against colourless to yellow background.

pH, temperature and time of heating affect the sensitivity of detection.

The reagent is suitable for silica gel, kieselguhr, cellulose, RP-8, RP-18 and modified (NH_2, CN, diol) layers.

The reagent is specific for detection of amino sugars.

23. 4-dimethylaminocinnamaldehyde–hydrochloric acid reagent

Spray solution : Dissolve 0.5 g of 4-dimethylaminocinnamaldehyde (PDAC) in 50 ml of 5 M hydrochloric acid and dilute to 100 ml with methanol.

Dilute with equal volume of methanol before use.

The solution may be stored in refrigerator for several days.

PDAC reacts with primary amines to yield coloured or fluorescent Schiff's base. After spraying, the chromatogram is heated to 100°C for 10 min. Coloured spots are obtained against colourless or yellow background. Greenish-yellow fluorescent spots are observed when examined under long wavelength (365 nm). The reagent is suitable for silica gel, cellulose and ion exchange layers. The reagent is used for detection of sulphonamides, primary amines and other drug substances such as bromhexine, ranitidine, orciprenaline, terbutaline, salbutamol, cephaloridine.

24. N,N-dimethyl-1,4-phenylene diamine reagent (Wurster's red reagent)

Spray solution : Dissolve 1 g of N,N-dimethyl-1,4-phenylene diamine dichloride (DPDD) in mixture containing 50 ml methanol, 50 ml water and 1 ml glacial acetic acid.

Store in refrigerator.

After removal of mobile phase, the chromatogram is sprayed with DPDD reagent and dried with cold air (to improve the contrast between coloured zones and the layer background, gentle warming of the chromatogram is recommended).

The reagent is suitable for silica gel and aluminium oxide layers.

The reagent can be used for detection of salbutamol, terbutaline, vitamin E, thiamine, paracetamol, thiourea, isoxsuperine, nylidrin, triamcinolone.

25. 2,4-dinitrophenylhydrazine reagent

Spray solution : Dissolve 50 mg of dinitrophenylhydrazine (DNPH) in methanol–conc. hydrochloric acid (90 + 10). The solution is stable for several days when stored in refrigerator.

DNPH reacts with carbonyl group of the drug molecule to yield hydrazone or osazones in the case of monosaccharides.

Warm the chromatogram in current of air to remove mobile phase and spray evenly with DNPH solution, followed by heating at 110°C for few minutes. Substances containing aldehyde or keto groups give yellow to orange spots against colourless background.

The reagent is suitable for silica gel and cellulose layers.

The reagent can be used for detection of corticosteroids (dexamethasone, beta-methasone, hydrocortisone, triamcinolone), nitrofurantoin, norfloxacin, ciprofloxacin, ofloxacin, pefloxacin, lomofloxacin, allantoin, paraformaldehyde, menadione.

26. Dithizone reagent

Spray solution : Dissolve 20 mg of dithizone in 100 ml of acetone. Store the solution in amber bottle in refrigerator.

Spray the chromatogram first with dithizone solution and then with 25% ammonia solution.

The reagent can be used for detection of cations such as zinc, copper, mercury, nickel, lead, iron, cobalt, cadmium, bismuth.

27. Dragendorff's reagent

Spray solution :

(a) Dissolve 1.7 g of basic bismuth nitrate and 20 g of tartaric acid in 80 ml of water.

(b) 40% w/v solution of potassium iodide in water.

Both the solutions are stable for several weeks when stored in refrigerator. Mix solutions (a) and (b) (1 : 1) just before use.

This reagent is most commonly used for detection of alkaloids. It may be used for detection of other nitrogenous compounds such as local anaesthetics (lignocaine, amethocaine), anti-histamines (pheniramine hydroxyzine, diphenylpyraline, chlorpheniramine, cyclizine), tranquillizers (diazepam, chlordiazepoxide, nitrazepam, imipramine, selegiline), phenylbutazone, oxyphenbutazone, phenylephrine, loperamide.

28. Ethanolamine diphenylborate reagent (Flavone reagent)

Spray solution : 1% w/v solution of ethanolamine diphenylborate in methanol.

The solution is stable for several days when stored in refrigerator. After spraying the reagent, chromatogram is sprayed with solution of liquid paraffin in n-hexane (1 + 2) or 5% methanolic solution of polyethylene glycol-4000 to stabilize the fluorescent spots. The plate may be examined after 30 min for full intensity of fluorescent spots.

The reagent is suitable for silica gel, kieselguhr, cellulose, RP-8, RP-18, polyamide and NH_2 layers.

The reagent is used for detection of flavonoids such as rutin, quercetin, kaempferol, hespiridine, carbohydrate (glucose, fructose, lactose).

29. Fluorescamine reagent

Spray solution :

(a) 0.1 mg/ml solution of fluorescamine (4-phenyl-spiro [furan-2-(H),1-phthalyl-3,3-dione]) in acetone.

(b) 10% solution of triethylamine in dichloromethane.

The chromatogram is dried at 110°C, cooled and sprayed evenly with solution (a), then air-dried for few seconds, followed by spraying with solution (b). Blue-green fluorescent spots appear against dark background when examined at long wavelength (365 nm). Triethylamine stabilizes the fluorescence.

The reagent is suitable for silica gel, kieselguhr and cellulose layers.

The reagent is used for detection of amino acids, primary amines (sulphonamides, catecholamines, gentamycin), peptides.

30. Formaldehyde–sulphuric acid reagent (Marquis' reagent)

Spray solution : Prepare solution of formaldehyde (37%) in conc. sulphuric acid (1 : 10).

Dipping solution : Add 10 ml of conc. sulphuric acid (> 98%) to 90 ml of ice-cooled methanol. To this, add 2 ml of formaldehyde (37%).

Both the solutions are stable for several weeks when stored in refrigerator.

Use current of air to remove the mobile phase, then immerse the plate in dipping solution for 3-4 s or spray evenly and then heat at 110°C for 15-20 min (dipping technique is recommended as, during spraying of the reagent, irritation of respiratory tract is often encountered.

The reagent is suitable for silica gel, kieselguhr and aluminium oxide layers. The reagent is used for detection of opium alkaloids (morphine, codeine, heroin), phenothiazine, β-blockers (acebutalol, propranolol, atenolol, alprenolol, dihydrazine). Other common drug substances which can be detected with Marquis' reagent are amtriptylene, atropine, chlordiazepoxide, chlorpheniramine, chlorpromazine, cyclizine, dextropropoxyphene, diazepam, diphenhydramine, diphenoxylate, ephedrine, hyoscine, imipramine, lignocaine, meclozine, mephenesin, guaiphenesin, mepyramine, naphazoline, phenylpropanolamine, selegiline.

31. Hydrochloric acid vapour reagent

Reagent solution : Place 10 ml of conc. sulphuric acid (98%) in a twin-trough chamber. Add carefully and dropwise 2 ml of conc. hydrochloric acid (> 37%) (if twin-trough chamber is not available, then use deep petri dish).

Reagent is to be prepared freshly.

The chromatogram, after it is free from mobile phase, is exposed to acid vapours by placing it in the chamber for 5 min and examined immediately both under short wavelengths UV (254 nm) and long wavelengths UV (365 nm). The reagent is suitable for silica gel, kieselguhr, RP-9 and RP-18 layers.

Note : The intensity of fluorescent spots can be increased by dipping the chromatogram in solution of liquid paraffin in n-hexane or chloroform (1 : 3).

The reagent is used for detection of digitalis glycosides, carbohydrates, opium alkaloids (papaverine, morphine, codeine, thebaine), barbiturates, diazepam, carbamezepine, phenytoin.

32.   Hydroxylamine–iron (III) chloride reagent

Spray solution :

(a) 2% solution of ferric chloride in 1% hydrochloric acid.

(b) 7% solution of hydroxylamine chloride in methanol.

(c) 7.0% solution of potassium hydroxide in methanol.

Mix solution (b) and (c) 1 : 1 to prepare hydroxylamine reagent.

Air-dry the chromatogram and first spray with hydroxylamine reagent followed by ferric chloride solution. Spots of different colours are observed.

The reagent is used for detection of amides, lactones, anhydrides, preservatives.

33.   8-hydroxyquinoline reagent

Spray solution : 0.5% solution of 8-hydroxyquinoline in methanol.

The solution can be stored for several days at room temperature.

The chromatogram is air-dried to remove mobile phase and then sprayed with the solution and exposed to ammonia (25%) vapours placed in twin-trough chamber for 5 min and immediately examine under UV light (254 nm or 365 nm). Mainly yellow spots are observed.

The reagent is used for detection of various cations : Mg^{2+}, Ca^{2+}, Sr^{2+}, Ba^{2+}, Fe^{2+}, Al^{3+}, Co^{2+}, Cu^{2+}, Bi^{2+}, Zn^{2+}, Cd^{2+}, Hg^{2+}.

Note : Coloured spots fluoresce when examined under long wavelength UV (365 nm).

34.   Iodine reagent

Iodine is non-specific universal non-destructive reagent for most of the unsaturated organic compounds. Detection by iodine involves physical concentration of iodine molecule in the lipophilic zones of the chromatogram without any chemical reaction. Iodine is strongly enriched in the substance zone than in the neighbouring polar substance-free portion of the layer. After treatment with iodine, brown spots with yellow background are obtained. Documentation should be carried out immediately as adsorbed iodine evaporates leading to almost fading of spots. If the iodine so adsorbed is allowed to completely evaporate, the same chromatogram can be subjected to other detection techniques as well as re-chromatographed (spots obtained with iodine can be stabilized by spraying the chromatogram with starch solution; resulting blue spots remain stable for long time).

Although iodine is fairly an inert halogen as compared to bromine and does not normally react with the substances that have been chromatographed, however, there are examples where irreversible chemical changes have been observed such as aromatic hydrocarbons, isoquinoline alkaloids and electrophilic substitutions and additions.

Following drug substances are reported to react with iodine, the reaction being irreversible : aspirin, ascorbic acid, hydrocortisone, analgin, benzocaine, isoniazid, para-cetamol, glycine, papaverine, piperazine, salicylic acid, sulphaguanidine, salicylamide, resorcinol, thymol. In case of phenolic steroids and morphine, iodine produces irreversible derivatization. In case of thiamine, there is oxidation of sulphur and attack on double bond in thiazole ring. Ethambutol, a poor UV-absorbing compound, reacts with iodine to form a chelate by ion-transfer, leading to a highly UV-absorbing compound. Best results are often obtained by dipping the chromatogram in iodine solution (0.1 to 0.25% in chloroform–methanol 1 : 1) than exposing to iodine vapours. Interestingly, molecular iodine is a strong quencher and must be removed before substances are examined under long UV (365 nm) for fluorescent properties of the compounds such as emetine and cephaeline.

35. Iodine vapour reagent

Place few crystals of iodine at the bottom of chromatographic chamber which can be tightly sealed. Iodine vapourizes and distributes itself uniformly in the entire interior of the chamber. Commercial iodine chambers are available with thermostatic controls to control the vaporization of iodine (gentle warming accelerates vaporization).

Caution : Iodine chamber should always be stored in fume cupboard.

The chromatogram, after it is free from mobile phase, is exposed to iodine vapours. Usually, by exposing for 5-10 min, most of the spots are revealed. Substances which chemically react with iodine give colourless spots; otherwise, brown spots on yellow background are observed. Since iodine has fluorescence quenching property, iodine containing spots on a layer containing fluorescence indicator (F_{254}) appear as dark spots on yellow-green fluorescent background when viewed under short wavelength UV (254 nm).

Caution : While using starch solution (0.5% soluble starch in water) to fix the spots/zones coloured by iodine it should be ensured that remaining area of the TLC plate is almost free from iodine, otherwise the whole background shall be coloured blue. This is well-known iodine–starch complex which is stable for a long period. Often starch treatment produces white spots on blue background, probably as a result of iodine being consumed by chemical reaction with the substance present as spot/zone, leaving large quantity of iodine in the background to produce blue starch–iodine complex.

The reagent is suitable for silica gel, aluminium oxide, kieselguhr, cellulose, wettable RP-18 layers. Modified layers (CN, NH_2) are not suitable as iodine gets strongly bound to the whole layer which gets coloured. Layers containing starch as binding agents are also not suitable. The reagent can be used for detection of fatty acids, phospholipids, prostaglandins, steroids, carotenoids, purine derivatives (caffeine, theophylline).

36. Iron (III) chloride reagent

Spray solution : Dissolve 0.5 g of iron (III) chloride in 2-3 ml of water and dilute to 50 ml with methanol or dilute hydrochloric acid.

The reagent is stable for several weeks if stored in refrigerator.

Remove the mobile phase with the aid of warm air and spray the chromatogram uniformly with the spray solution and heat at 100-150°C for 5-10 min. Coloured spots against pale-yellow background are observed. Flavones appear as red to violet, flavonoid glycosides as green/wine red/red/blue-violet, phenothiazines as pink, salicylates as pink, inorganic anions (nitrite, iodate, chromate, vanadate, selenite, selenate) as pale yellow to blue green. The reagent can be employed on silica gel, kieselguhr, cellulose and polyamide layers. Most common drug substances which can be detected with the reagent are aspirin, paracetamol, morphine, ergotamine, adrenaline, noradrenaline, diclofenac, PAS.

37. Iron (III) chloride–potassium ferricyanide reagent (Barton's reagent)

Spray solution :

(a) 1% solution of potassium ferricyanide in water.

(b) 2% solution of ferric chloride in water.

Immediately before use mix solutions (a) and (b) in equal proportion.

All the solutions as well as final spray solution should be stored in refrigerator.

After the mobile phase is removed, the chromatogram is sprayed evenly and then heated for 5-10 min at 110°C. Blue spots appear against colourless or pale-yellow background. Colour intensity of the spots can be enhanced if, at the end, chromatogram is sprayed with 2 M hydrochloric acid.

Note : After 15-20 min, the blue spots/zones tends to fade.

The reagent is suitable for silica gel, kieselguhr and cellulose layers.

The reagent may be used for detection of aromatic amines, phenols, phenolic steroids, ibuprofen, ketoprofen, diclofenac.

38. Isonicotinic acid hydrazide reagent (INH reagent)

Spray solution : Dissolve 0.4 g of isonicotinic acid hydrazide (isoniazid) in 100 ml of methanol, add 1 ml hydrochloric acid.

The chromatogram is first dried with cold air and then sprayed with the reagent and left at room temperature. Coloured hydrazones are formed which fluoresce on dark background when examined under long wavelength UV (365 nm). The treatment of the chromatogram with liquid paraffin–n-hexane (1 + 2) intensifies the fluorescence.

The reagent is suitable for silica gel, kieselguhr and cellulose layers.

The reagent is used for detection of diloxanide furoate, clobetasol, nitrofurantoin, spironolactone and ketosteroids.

39. 3-methyl-2-benzothiazolinone hydrazone reagent (MBTH reagent or Besthorn's reagent)

Spray solution : 0.5% solution of MBTH in methanol. Filter, if precipitates appear. Prepare fresh.

The chromatogram is freed from mobile phase and evenly sprayed with the spray solution and heated at 110-120°C for 2 hrs. Coloured spots against pale background are observed. The spots exhibit yellow to yellow-orange fluorescence in long wavelength UV (365 nm).

The reagent can be employed on silica gel, kieselguhr, cellulose and polyamide layers. The reagent is used for detection of methyldopa, paracetamol, ketoconazole, analgin, mephenesin, pyrazinamide, ethambutol, sulphadoxine, omeprazole, mycotoxins, aflatoxins and carbonyl compounds.

40. 1,2-naphthoquinone-4-sulphonic acid reagent (Folin's reagent)

Spray solution : Dissolve 0.25 g of 1,2-naphthoquinone-4-sulphonic acid, sodium salt in 5% aqueous sodium carbonate.

The chromatogram is freed from mobile phase by warm air and then sprayed with the solution evenly till the layer is transparent. Dry in stream of cold air. Coloured spots against yellow background are observed.

Note : It is possible to differentiate amino acids on the basis of colours of different shades. There are several modifications of this reagent depending on the class of compounds (aromatic amines, aliphatic amines, amino acids).

The reagent is suitable for silica gel, kieselguhr, aluminium oxide, polyamide and cellulose layers.

The reagent can be used for detection of amino acids, peptides, aromatic/aliphatic amines, ergot alkaloids, sulfones, sulfoxides, diuretics (chlorthalidone, hydrochlorothiazide) and other common drugs such as pyrimethamine, analgin, primaquine, folic acid, sulphalene, sulphadoxine, dapsone, piroxicam, metoclopramide, prochlorperazine, cimetidine.

41. Ninhydrin reagent

Spray solution : Dissolve 0.25 g of ninhydrin in 95 ml of isopropyl alcohol, add 5 ml of glacial acetic acid.

Remove the excess mobile phase from chromatogram with the aid of air current and then spray the reagent followed by spraying with copper nitrate reagent and heat at 110°C for 5 min. Reddish and bluish spots are observed on a pale background. The reagent is suitable for silica gel and cellulose layers.

The reagent is used for detection of amino acids, peptides, amines. Other common substances which can be detected with the reagent are gentamycin, ampicillin, ephedrine, pseudoephedrine, folic acid, methyldopa, diazepam, neomycin, diloxanide, naphazoline, cimetidine, lisinopril, pantothenic acid, pyrazinamide, primaquine, promethazine, phenylpropanolamine.

42. Nitric acid vapours

Fuming nitric acid is used as the reagent.

The chromatogram freed from mobile phase is placed with layer down in chamber containing fuming nitric acid for 1-2 min. It is then freed of excess nitrous fumes with the help of cold air and then heated. Aromatic compounds generally give yellow to brown spots which fluoresce when examined under long wavelength (365 nm).

Note : Fuming nitric acid being highly corrosive, it is advisable to use mixture of 50% nitric acid and 2 M hydrochloric acid to generate nitrous fumes. Use of sodium nitrite and sulphuric acid is also recommended.

The reagent is suitable for wide range of TLC layers such as silica gel, kieselguhr, aluminium oxide, cellulose, chiral, RP-8, RP-18 and modified (NH_2, CN, diol) and impregnated ($AgNO_3$) layers.

The reagent is used for detection of ephedrine, pseudoephedrine, xanthene derivatives, diazepam, testosterone, sugars, phospholipids, imipramine.

43. Perchloric acid reagent

Spray solution : Add perchloric acid carefully to 50 ml of water, cool and dilute to 100 ml with methanol.

For steroids, usually 2% solution is employed, whereas for detection of bile salts, 5% solution is recommended. After the chromatogram is freed from mobile phase, it is sprayed with the reagent and heated at 80°C for 30 min. Coloured spots are observed on colourless background. These spots fluoresce when examined under long wavelength UV (365 nm).

Caution :

1. Do not heat for longer time as it can lead to charring of substances.
2. As perchloric acid is explosive, dipping is recommended.
3. Heating should be carried in fume cupboard having efficient exhaust system to avoid explosion.
4. The reagent is suitable for silica gel and kieselguhr layers.

The reagent can be used for detection of steroids, bile salts, antiepileptics (carbamezepine), barbiturates, fatty acids, sugars and tranquilizers (diazepam, chlordiazepoxide).

44. Phosphomolybdic acid reagent

Spray solution : 1% solution of the acid in methanol.

The solution is stable for several days when stored in amber-coloured bottles. Phosphomolybdic acid acts as oxidizing agent and in the process gets reduced to Mo (IV) which forms blue complex with excess of Mo (VI).

After drying the chromatogram with warm air, it is sprayed with the solution till the layer is yellow. Heat to 120°C briefly. Blue spots against yellow background appear.

Note : Brief heating is usually recommended for optimal colour development. Prolonged heating results in background being darkened.

The reagent is suitable for silica gel, aluminium oxide, polyamide, cellulose, RP-2 and RP-18 layers as well as impregnated ($AgNO_3$) layers.

The reagent is used for detection of morphine, codeine, thymol, menthol, eugenol, carvone, ergot alkaloids, bile acids, vitamin E, ascorbic acid, fatty acids, prostaglandins, lipids, steroids.

45. Potassium dichromate–sulphuric acid reagent (Chromosulphuric acid reagent)

Spray solution : 5% solution of potassium dichromate in 30% sulphuric acid.

It is a destructive universal visualization reagent. After the chromatogram is dried, it is sprayed with the reagent and plate is allowed to dry in the air for 15 min. Substances appear as coloured spots against yellowish-green background. To aid visualization, heating may sometime be required. The reagent is suitable for silica gel, kieselguhr, RP-8, RP-18, polyamide, cellulose and modified (CN, NH_2, diol) layers.

The reagent is used for detection of almost all organic compounds giving different colours : imipramine, antazoline, bromhexine, atropine, atenolol, bisacodyl, cimetidine, codeine, caffeine, cyproheptadine, dextromethorphan, dextropropoxyphene, diphenhydramine, promethazine, trifluoperazine, triflupromazine, haloperidol, pheniramine, glycerin, ethylene glycol, diethylene glycol, propylglycol.

46. Potassium ferricyanide–sodium hydroxide reagent (Alkaline potassium ferricyanide reagent)

Spray solution : Dissolve 10 mg of potassium ferricyanide and 1 g sodium hydroxide in 5 ml of water and dilute to 20 ml with methanol.

Prepare just before use.

The solution can be used as spray reagent as well as for dipping.

The chromatogram is air-dried to remove the mobile phase, sprayed and again air-dried. Orange to blue fluorescent spots are observed when examined under long wavelength (365 nm).

The reagent is suitable for silica gel, kieselguhr and cellulose layers.

The reagent is used for detection of thiamine, adrenaline, noradrenaline, isoprenaline, dopa, methyldopa, febendazole.

47. Potassium permanganate–sulphuric acid reagent (Acidified potassium permanganate reagent)

Spray solution : 1% solution of potassium permanganate in 0.25 M sulphuric acid.

The reagent is used for detection of ephedrine, ethambutol, benzyl nicotinate, ethyl nicotinate, methyl nicotinate, buclosamide, broxyquinoline, frusemide, indomethacin, lorazepam, methocarbamol, metronidazole, neomycin paracetamol, phenazopyridine, phenazone, phenylephrine, propyphenazone, pseudoephedrine, pyridoxine, reserpine, rifampicin, salbutamol, salicylamide, salicylic acid, streptomycin, terbutaline.

48. Sulphuric acid reagent

Spray solution : Cautiously add 10 ml of conc. sulphuric acid to 90 ml of ice-cooled methanol placed in freezing mixture.

It is a universal reagent and almost all classes of compounds can be detected by charring at elevated temperature. The production of coloured spots or their fluorescent behaviour depend on the duration of heating.

The chromatogram is air-dried and then evenly sprayed, dried and heated at 105°C for 30 min. Usually dark brown spots appear as a result of charring. However, when examined under long wavelength (365 nm), yellow, green, red or blue fluorescent spots are observed.

The reagent is suitable for silica gel, kieselguhr and RP layers.

The reagent is used for detection of vitamin A, aflatoxins, phenothiazines, carotene, cardiac glycosides, prostaglandins, ethinyl estradiol, spironolactone.

49.   Sulphanilic acid, diazotized reagent (Pauly's reagent)

Spray solution :

(a) 5% solution of sodium nitrite in water.

(b) Dissolve 5 g of sulphanilic acid in 5 ml conc. hydrochloric acid with gentle warming and dilute to 500 ml with water.

(c) 10% solution of sodium carbonate in water.

While cooling, mix 10 ml of solution (a) with 10 ml of solution (b), keep in ice-bath for 15 min. Immediately before use, to this add 20 ml of solution (c).

Spray solution should be prepared fresh. Diazotized sulphanilic acid couples with aromatic amines and phenol to yield azo dye.

After the chromatogram is freed from mobile phase, it is sprayed with freshly prepared diazotized solution until the layer is transparent. Coloured spots appear against colourless background which are quite stable. The reagent is suitable for silica gel, kieselguhr and cellulose layers. The reagent is used for detection of sulphonamides, phenols, preservatives, flavonoids, cumarins, histamine, clotrimazole, tinidazole, metronidazole, carboxylic acids (sorbic acid, malic acid, citric acid).

50.   Vanillin–sulphuric acid reagent

Spray solution : 1% solution of vanillin in 5% methanolic sulphuric acid.
Prepare fresh.

The chromatogram is first dried in stream of cold water and evenly sprayed with spray solution. The plate is heated to 105°C for 5 min. Different coloured spots (yellow to dark violet) appear on heating against light background. Fluorescent spots are seen when examined under long wavelength UV (365 nm). The reagent can be employed on silica gel, kieselguhr, RP-8 and RP-18 layers.

The reagent is used for detection of steroids, prostaglandins, carbohydrates, cardiac glycosides, antibiotics, mycotoxins, essential oil components (menthol, thymol, carophylline), other common drugs (paracetamol, analgin, amoxycillin, isoniazid, benzocaine, promethazine, chlorthalidone).

Cardiovascular System

- β-blockers
- Antiarrhythmic drugs
- Antianginal drugs
- Anti-hypertensive drugs
- Diuretics

53

PROTOCOLS OF A THIN LAYER CHROMATOGRAM

Chromatogram No. 1

Formulation : Propranolol hydrochloride, Hydrochlorothiazide
Classification : Cardiac drugs
Dosage form : Tablets
Standard solution : Working standard of each drug substance was dissolved in methanol.
Sample solution : Sample was extracted with methanol, centrifuged for application.
Chromatographic conditions :

Test plate : TLC pre-coated plate, silica gel 60F$_{254}$ (E. Merck)

Format : 10 × 10 cm *Thickness :* 250 mm

Volume spotted : 10 µl *Separation technique :* Ascending

Mobile phase : Toluene–methanol–ethyl acetate–ammonia (80 + 20 + 10 + 02, v/v)

Chamber saturation : 20 min *Migration distance :* 100 mm

Detection : UV (short) and in situ spectra/iodine vapours

HRf :	Propranolol hydrochloride	20
	Trimethoprim (IS)	35
	Hydrochlorothiazide	45

Comments : —
Reference : —

PROTOCOLS OF A THIN LAYER CHROMATOGRAM

Chromatogram No. 2

Formulation : Propranolol hydrochloride, Hydrochlorothiazide
Classification : Cardiac drugs
Dosage form : Tablets
Standard solution : See Chromatogram No. 1.
Sample solution : See Chromatogram No. 1.
Chromatographic conditions :

    Test plate : Hand-made plate, silica gel GF$_{254}$

    Format : 10×20 cm   *Thickness :* About 250 μm

    Volume spotted : 10 μl   *Separation technique :* Ascending

    Mobile phase : Chloroform–methanol–ammonia (90 + 10 + 0.4, v/v)

    Chamber saturation : 30 min   *Migration distance :* 150 mm

    Detection : UV (short) or iodine vapours

    HRf :   Hydrochlorothiazide   15

            Propranolol hydrochloride   50

Comments : —
Reference : —

PROTOCOLS OF A THIN LAYER CHROMATOGRAM

Chromatogram No. 3

Formulation : Propranolol hydrochloride, Hydrochlorothiazide

Classification : Cardiac drugs

Dosage form : Tablets

Standard solution : See Chromatogram No. 1.

Sample solution : See Chromatogram No. 1.

Chromatographic conditions :

Test plate : Hand-made TLC plate, silica gel 60F$_{254}$, impregnated with 5% silicone oil in light petroleum ether for reversed-phase characteristics

Format : 5 × 20 cm   *Thickness :* About 250 µm

Volume spotted : 10 µl   *Separation technique :* Ascending

Mobile phase : 0.5 M sodium chloride–methanol–glacial acetic acid (120 + 80 + 0.1, v/v)

Chamber saturation : 45 min   *Migration distance :* 150 mm

Detection : UV (short)

HRf :   Propranolol hydrochloride   30

        Hydrochlorothiazide   55

Comments : As a result of chromatography being performed in reversed-phase, Rf values get reversed as compared to normal-phase chromatography (see Chromatogram No. 2).

Reference : —

PROTOCOLS OF A THIN LAYER CHROMATOGRAM

Chromatogram No. 4

Formulation : Propranolol hydrochloride, Hydroflumethiazide

Classification : Cardiac drugs

Dosage form : Tablets

Standard solution : Working standard of each drug substance was dissolved in methanol.

Sample solution : Powdered sample was extracted with methanol in ultrasonic water bath (5 min), centrifuged, supernatant used for

Chromatographic conditions :

Test plate : Hand-made TLC plate, silica gel GF$_{254}$ (activated at 105°C for 30 min and cooled prior to use)

Format : 10 × 20 cm   *Thickness :* 250 μm

Volume spotted : 10 μl   *Separation technique :* Ascending

Mobile phase :   1. Toluene–methanol–ammonia (75 + 25 + 0.5, v/v)

2. Butyl acetate–formic acid–chloroform (60 + 40 + 20, v/v)

3. Methanol–ammonia (200 + 03, v/v)

Chamber saturation : 30 min   *Migration distance :* 150 mm

Detection : UV (short)/iodine vapours

HRf :	1	2	3
Hydroflumethiazide	10	90	70
Propranolol hydrochloride	30	70	35

Comments : —

Reference : —

PROTOCOLS OF A THIN LAYER CHROMATOGRAM

Chromatogram No. 5

Formulation : Reserpine, Chlorthalidone

Classification : Cardiac drugs

Dosage form : Tablets

Standard solution : Working standard of each drug substance was dissolved in chloroform for spotting.

Sample solution : Powdered sample was extracted with chloroform, supernatant used for spotting.

Chromatographic conditions :

Test plate : Handmade TLC plate, silica gel GF$_{254}$ (activate for 105°C for 30 min prior to use)

Format : 10 × 20 cm   *Thickness :* 250 µm

Volume spotted : 10 µl   *Separation technique :* Ascending

Mobile phase :   1. Toluene–methanol–ammonia (75 + 25 + 0.25, v/v)

                          2. Toluene–ethyl acetate–acetone–ammonia (50 + 25 + 25 + 0.2, v/v)

Chamber saturation : 20 min   *Migration distance :* 150 mm

Detection : UV (short), iodine vapour

HRf :

	1	2
Chlorthalidone	30	35
Reserpine	65	85

Comments : —

Reference : —

PROTOCOLS OF A THIN LAYER CHROMATOGRAM

Chromatogram No. 6

Formulation : Metoprolol tartrate, Hydrochlorothiazide

Classification : Cardiac drugs

Dosage form : Tablets

Standard solution : Working standard of both the drug substances was dissolved in methanol for spotting.

Sample solution : The powdered sample was extracted with methanol, centrifuged and supernatant used for spotting.

Chromatographic conditions :

Test plate : Handmade TLC plates, silica gel F_{254} (activate at 105°C for 30 min prior to use)

Format : 10×20 cm   *Thickness :* 250 μm

Volume spotted : 10 μl   *Separation technique :* Ascending

Mobile phase : 1. Chloroform–methanol–ammonia (90 + 10 + 0.5, v/v)

2. Toluene–methanol–ammonia (75 + 25 + 0.25, v/v)

3. Toluene–ethyl acetate–acetone–ammonia (50 + 25 + 25 + 0.2, v/v)

Chamber saturation : 20 min   *Migration distance :* 150 mm

Detection : Iodine vapours

HRf :	1	2	3
Hydrochlorothiazide	15	20	25
Metoprolol tartrate	30	10	10

Comments : —

Reference : —

PROTOCOLS OF A THIN LAYER CHROMATOGRAM

Formulation : Reserpine, Dihydralazine sulphate, Hydrochlorothiazide

Classification : Cardiac drugs

Dosage form : Tablets

Standard solution : Working standard of all the drug substances was dissolved in methanol for spotting.

Sample solution : The powdered sample was extracted with methanol in ultrasonic bath (5 min), centrifuged and used for spotting.

Chromatographic conditions :

Test plate : Handmade TLC plates, coated with silica gel GF_{254} (activate at 105°C for 30 min prior to use)

Format : 10 × 20 cm   *Thickness :* 250 μm

Volume spotted : 10 μl   *Separation technique :* Ascending

Mobile phase : Toluene–methanol–ammonia (75 + 25 + 0.25, v/v)

Chamber saturation : 30 min   *Migration distance :* 150 mm

Detection : UV, iodine vapours

HRf : Hydrochlorothiazide   20

         Dihydralazine sulphate   45

         Reserpine   65

Comments : —

Reference : —

PROTOCOLS OF A THIN LAYER CHROMATOGRAM

Chromatogram No. 8

Formulation : Acebutalol hydrochloride, Hydrochlorothiazide

Classification : Cardiac drugs

Dosage form : Tablets

Standard solution : Dissolve appropriate quantity of working standard of each drug substance in methanol and use the solution for spotting.

Sample solution : The powdered sample is extracted with methanol in ultrasonic water bath (5 min), centrifuged, supernatant used for spotting.

Chromatographic conditions :

Test plate : TLC pre-coated plate, silica gel $60F_{254}$, aluminium (E. Merck)

Format : 10×10 cm *Thickness :* 250 μm

Volume spotted : 10 μl *Separation technique :* Ascending

Mobile phase : Toluene–n-propanol–ammonia (60 + 40 + 0.5, v/v)

Chamber saturation : 30 min *Migration distance :* 70 mm

Detection : UV (short)

HRf : Acebutalol hydrochloride   10

        Hydrochlorothiazide   50

Comments : —

Reference : —

PROTOCOLS OF A THIN LAYER CHROMATOGRAM

Chromatogram No. 9

Formulation : Acebutalol hydrochloride, Hydrochlorothiazide

Classification : Cardiac drugs

Dosage form : Tablets

Standard solution : See Chromatogram No. 8

Sample solution : See Chromatogram No. 8

Chromatographic conditions :

Test plate : TLC pre-coated plate, silica gel 60F$_{254}$ impregnated with 5% silicone oil in n-hexane for reversed-phase characteristics

Format : 10 × 10 cm   *Thickness :* 250 μm

Volume spotted : 10 μl   *Separation technique :* Ascending

Mobile phase : 0.5 M Sodium chloride–methanol–acetonitrile–glacial acetic acid (50 + 20 + 30 + 01, v/v)

Chamber saturation : 30 min   *Migration distance :* 70 mm

Detection : UV (short)

HRf :   Acebutalol hydrochloride   25

       Hydrochlorothiazide   75

Comments : —

Reference : —

PROTOCOLS OF A THIN LAYER CHROMATOGRAM

Chromatogram No. 10

Formulation : Acebutalol, Propranolol, Atenolol, Dihydralazine

Classification : Cardiac drugs

Dosage form : Tablets

Standard solution : Dissolve each drug substance in methanol for spotting.

Sample solution : Suspend the powdered sample in water, make alkaline and extract with diethyl ether–dichloromethane (4 + 1), evaporate to dryness and dissolve the residue in methanol.

Chromatographic conditions :

Test plate : TLC pre-coated plate (plastic), SIL N-HR 254 nm (M & N)

Format : 5 × 20 cm   *Thickness :* 250 μm

Volume spotted : 10 μl   *Separation technique :* Ascending

Mobile phase : Ethylacetate–methanol–aqueous ammonia (8 + 1 + 1, v/v)

Chamber saturation :   *Migration distance :* 80 mm

Detection : UV-254 nm or spray with conc. sulphuric acid followed by detection by UV.

HRf :   Dihydralazine   00
          Atenolol   54
          Acebutalol   73
          Propranolol   81

Comments : —

Reference : TLC Application Notes (M & N), p. A-20.

PROTOCOLS OF A THIN LAYER CHROMATOGRAM

Formulation : Clonidine hydrochloride, Hydrochlorothiazide

Classification : Cardiac drugs

Dosage form : Tablets

Standard solution : Appropriate quantity of working standard of both the drug substance is dissolved in methanol for spotting.

Sample solution : Extract the powdered sample with methanol in ultrasonic water bath (10 min), centrifuge and use for spotting.

Chromatographic conditions :

Test plate : TLC pre-coated plate, silica gel $60F_{254}$/Hand-made TLC plate silica gel GF_{254} (activate at 105° for 30 min prior to use)

Format : 10 × 20 cm   *Thickness :* 250 µm

Volume spotted : 10 µl   *Separation technique :* Ascending

Mobile phase :   1. Toluene–acetone–ammonia (50 + 50 + 01, v/v)
                   2. Toluene–methanol–ammonia (75 + 25 + 0.25, v/v)

Chamber saturation : 30 min   *Migration distance :* 150 mm

Detection : UV (short), iodine vapours or spray with Dragendorff's reagent

HRf :	1	2
Hydrochlorothiazide	40	20
Clonidine HCl	60	45

Comments : —

Reference : —

PROTOCOLS OF A THIN LAYER CHROMATOGRAM

Chromatogram No. 12

Formulation : Amiloride hydrochloride, Hydrochlorothiazide

Classification : Cardiac drugs

Dosage form : Tablets

Standard solution : Appropriate quantity of the each working standard is taken up in methanol for application.

Sample solution : Extract powdered sample in methanol in ultrasonic water bath (5 min), centrifuge and use for spotting.

Chromatographic conditions :

Test plate : TLC pre-coated plate, silica gel 60F$_{254}$

Format : 10 × 20 cm   *Thickness :* 250 μm

Volume spotted : 10 μl   *Separation technique :* Ascending

Mobile phase :   1. Chloroform–methanol–ammonia (75 + 25 + 02, v/v)

                        2. Ethyl acetate–methanol–ammonia (75 + 10 + 08, v/v)

Chamber saturation : 30 min   *Migration distance :* 100 mm

Detection : UV

HRf :	1	2
Amiloride hydrochloride	20	45
Hydrochlorothiazide	60	65

Comments : —

Reference : —

PROTOCOLS OF A THIN LAYER CHROMATOGRAM

Chromatogram No. 13

Formulation : Amiloride hydrochloride, Hydrochlorothiazide

Classification : Cardiac drugs

Dosage form : Tablets

Standard solution : See Chromatogram No. 12.

Sample solution : See Chromatogram No. 12.

Chromatographic conditions :

Test plate : TLC pre-coated plate, silica gel 60F$_{254}$ impregnated with 5% silicone oil in petroleum ether (40-60)

Format : 10 × 10 cm   *Thickness :* 250 μm

Volume spotted : 10 μl   *Separation technique :* Ascending

Mobile phase : 0.5 M Sodium chloride–methanol–glacial acetic acid (12 + 08 + 0.01, v/v)

Chamber saturation : —   *Migration distance :* 70 mm

Detection : UV (short)

HRf : Amiloride hydrochloride   15

      Hydrochlorothiazide   70

Comments : —

Reference : —

PROTOCOLS OF A THIN LAYER CHROMATOGRAM

Chromatogram No. 14

Formulation : Amiloride hydrochloride, Furosemide

Classification : Cardiac drugs

Dosage form : Tablets

Standard solution : Dissolve appropriate quantity of each drug drug substance in methanol for application.

Sample solution : Extract powdered sample with methanol in ultrasonic water bath (5 min), decant and use the supernatant for spotting.

Chromatographic conditions :

Test plate : TLC pre-coated plate, silica gel 60F$_{254}$

Format : 10 × 10 cm   *Thickness :* 250 μm

Volume spotted : 10 μl   *Separation technique :* Ascending

Mobile phase : 1. Chloroform–methanol–glacial acetic acid (85 + 15 + 0.5, v/v)

2. Chloroform–methanol–glacial acetic acid (90 + 5 + 5, v/v)

3. Chloroform–methanol–glacial acetic acid (90 + 50 + 50, v/v)

4. Ethyl acetate–methanol–ammonia (75 + 10 + 08, v/v)

Chamber saturation : 30 min   *Migration distance :* 70 mm

Detection : UV (short)

HRf :

	1	2	3	4
Amiloride hydrochloride	15	07	05	45
Furosemide	35	32	32	15

Comments : These mobile phases are suitable for detection of impurities in furosemide.

Reference : —

PROTOCOLS OF A THIN LAYER CHROMATOGRAM

Chromatogram No. 15

Formulation : Spironolactone, Hydroflumethiazide

Classification : Cardiac drugs

Dosage form : Tablets

Standard solution : Dissolve appropriate quantity of working standard of both the drug substances in methanol with the aid of sonication for application.

Sample solution : Suspend powdered sample in methanol, sonicate for 5 min, centrifuge and use for spotting.

Chromatographic conditions :

Test plate : TLC pre-coated plate, silica gel 60F254 or hand-made plate silica gel GF254

Format : 10 × 20 cm   *Thickness :* 250 μm

Volume spotted : 10 μl   *Separation technique :* Ascending

Mobile phase :   1. n-hexane–ethyl acetate–glacial acetic acid (50 + 50 + 0.5, v/v)

2. Toluene–methanol–ammonia (75 + 25 + 0.25, v/v)

3. Butyl acetate–formic acid–chloroform (60 + 40 + 20, v/v)

4. Chloroform–methanol (90 + 10, v/v)

Chamber saturation : 30 min   *Migration distance :* 150 mm

Detection : UV (short)

HRf :

	1	2	3	4
Spironolactone	55	75	75	70
Hydroflumethiazide	20	10	60	10

Comments : —

Reference : —

PROTOCOLS OF A THIN LAYER CHROMATOGRAM

Chromatogram No. 16

Formulation : Spironolactone, Hydroflumethiazide

Classification : Cardiac drugs

Dosage form : Tablets

Standard solution : See Chromatogram No. 15.

Sample solution : See Chromatogram No. 15.

Chromatographic conditions :

Test plate : TLC pre-coated plate, silica gel 60F$_{254}$ impregnated with 5% silicone oil in petroleum ether 40-60

Format : 10 × 10 cm   *Thickness :* 250 μm

Volume spotted : 10 μl   *Separation technique :* Ascending

Mobile phase : 0.5 M sodium chloride–methanol–acetonitrile–glacial acetic acid (50 + 20 + 30 + 01, v/v)

Chamber saturation : —   *Migration distance :* 70 mm

Detection : UV (short)

HRf :   Spironolactone   25

      Hydroflumethiazide   70

Comments : Note for reversal of Rf values as compared to normal-phase chromatography.

Reference : —

PROTOCOLS OF A THIN LAYER CHROMATOGRAM

Chromatogram No. 17

Formulation : Captopril, Hydrochlorothiazide

Classification : Cardiac drugs

Dosage form : Tablets

Standard solution : Dissolve working standard of both the drug substances in methanol for application.

Sample solution : Extract the powdered sample with methanol by sonication, centrifuge and use for spotting.

Chromatographic conditions :

Test plate : TLC pre-coated plate, silica gel 60F$_{254}$

Format : 10 × 10 cm   *Thickness :* 250 μm

Volume spotted : 10 μl   *Separation technique :* Ascending

Mobile phase : Chloroform–methanol–ammonia (80 + 20 + 02, v/v)

Chamber saturation : 30 min   *Migration distance :* 70 mm

Detection : UV (short) or iodine vapours

HRf : Captopril   15

       Hydrochlorothiazide   25

Comments : —

Reference : —

PROTOCOLS OF A THIN LAYER CHROMATOGRAM

Chromatogram No. 18

Formulation : Enalapril maleate, Hydrochlorothiazide

Classification : Cardiac drugs

Dosage form : Tablets

Standard solution : See Chromatogram No. 17.

Sample solution : See Chromatogram No. 17.

Chromatographic conditions :

Test plate : TLC pre-coated plate, silica gel $60F_{254}$

Format : 10 × 10 cm   *Thickness :* 250 μm

Volume spotted : 10 μl   *Separation technique :* Ascending

Mobile phase : Chloroform–methanol–glacial acetic acid (85 + 15 + 01, v/v)

Chamber saturation : 30 min   *Migration distance :* 70 mm

Detection : UV (short) or iodine vapours

HRf : Enalapril maleate   15

      Hydrochlorothiazide   55

Comments : —

Reference : —

PROTOCOLS OF A THIN LAYER CHROMATOGRAM

Chromatogram No. 19

Formulation : Atenolol, Chlorthalidone

Classification : Cardiac drugs

Dosage form : Tablets

Standard solution : Solution of both the drug substances is prepared in methanol for spotting.

Sample solution : Extract powdered sample with methanol by sonication, decant and use supernatant liquid for spotting.

Chromatographic conditions :

Test plate : TLC pre-coated plate, silica gel 60F$_{254}$

Format : 10 × 10 cm   *Thickness :* 250 μm

Volume spotted : 10 μl   *Separation technique :* Ascending

Mobile phase : Toluene–iso-propanol–ammonia (65 + 35 + 0.2, v/v)

Chamber saturation : —   *Migration distance :* 70 mm

Detection : UV (short) or iodine vapours

HRf : Atenolol   10

   Chlorthalidone   55

Comments : —

Reference : —

PROTOCOLS OF A THIN LAYER CHROMATOGRAM

Chromatogram No. 20

Formulation : Atenolol, Chlorthalidone

Classification : Cardiac drugs

Dosage form : Tablets

Standard solution : See Chromatogram No. 19.

Sample solution : See Chromatogram No. 19.

Chromatographic conditions :

Test plate : Hand-made TLC plate, silica gel GF_{254} impregnated with 5% silicone oil in petroleum ether (40-60)

Format : 10 × 10 cm   *Thickness :* 250 μm

Volume spotted : 10 μl   *Separation technique :* Ascending

Mobile phase : 0.5 M sodium chloride–ammonia–acetonitrile–glacial acetic acid (100 + 40 + 60 + 0.1, v/v)

Chamber saturation : —   *Migration distance :* 70 mm

Detection : UV (short) or iodine vapours

HRf :   Atenolol   35

　　　　Chlorthalidone   50

Comments : —

Reference : —

PROTOCOLS OF A THIN LAYER CHROMATOGRAM

Chromatogram No. 21

Formulation : Atenolol, Nifedipine

Classification : Cardiac drugs

Dosage form : Tablets

Standard solution : Prepare solution of both the drug substances in methanol for spotting.

Sample solution : Suspend powdered sample in methanol, sonicate for 10 min, centrifuge and use the clear solution for spotting.

Chromatographic conditions :

Test plate : TLC pre-coated plate, silica gel 60F$_{254}$

Format : 10 × 10 cm   *Thickness :* 250 μm

Volume spotted : 10 μl   *Separation technique :* Ascending

Mobile phase : Toluene–iso-propanol–ammonia (75 + 25 + 01, v/v)

Chamber saturation : 30 min   *Migration distance :* 70 mm

Detection : UV (short) or iodine vapours

HRf : Atenolol   10

       Nifedipine   70

Comments : —

Reference : —

PROTOCOLS OF A THIN LAYER CHROMATOGRAM

Chromatogram No. 22

Formulation : Atenolol, Nifedipine

Classification : Cardiac drugs

Dosage form : Tablets

Standard solution : See Chromatogram No. 21.

Sample solution : See Chromatogram No. 21.

Chromatographic conditions :

Test plate : Hand-made TLC plate, silica gel GF_{254} impregnated with silicone oil in petroleum ether (40-60)

Format : 10 × 10 cm   *Thickness :* 250 μm

Volume spotted : 10 μl   *Separation technique :* Ascending

Mobile phase : 0.5 M sodium chloride–ammonia–acetonitrile (50 + 20 + 30 + 01, v/v)

Chamber saturation : —   *Migration distance :* 70 mm

Detection : UV (short) or iodine vapours

HRf :   Atenolol   55

    Nifedipine   25

Comments : All experiments to be conducted in dark. See reversal of Rf values as compared to normal-phase chromatography (Chromatogram No. 21).

Reference : —

PROTOCOLS OF A THIN LAYER CHROMATOGRAM

Chromatogram No. 23

Formulation : Spironolactone, Furosemide

Classification : Cardiac drugs

Dosage form : Tablets

Standard solution : Dissolve working standard of each drug substance in methanol for spotting.

Sample solution : Extract powdered sample with methanol by sonication, centrifuge and use the clear liquid for spotting.

Chromatographic conditions :

Test plate : TLC pre-coated plate, silica gel 60F$_{254}$

Format : 10 × 10 cm   *Thickness :* 250 μm

Volume spotted : 10 μl   *Separation technique :* Ascending

Mobile phase :   1. n-hexane–ethyl acetate–glacial acetic acid (40 + 60 + 0.5, v/v)

2. Chloroform–methanol–glacial acetic acid (70 + 30 + 01, v/v)

3. Chloroform–ethyl acetate–glacial acetic acid (70 + 30 + 05, v/v)

Chamber saturation : —   *Migration distance :* 70 mm

Detection : UV (short) or iodine vapours

HRf :	1	2	3
Spironolactone	60	50	55
Furosemide	45	85	42

Comments : —

Reference : —

PROTOCOLS OF A THIN LAYER CHROMATOGRAM

Chromatogram No. 24

Formulation : Spironolactone, Furosemide

Classification : Cardiac drugs

Dosage form : Tablets

Standard solution : See Chromatogram No. 23.

Sample solution : See Chromatogram No. 23.

Chromatographic conditions :

Test plate : Hand-made TLC plate, silica gel GF_{254} impregnated with 5% silicone oil in petroleum ether

Format : 10 × 10 cm   *Thickness :* 250 μm

Volume spotted : 10 μl   *Separation technique :* Ascending

Mobile phase : 0.5 M sodium chloride–methanol–acetonitrile–glacial acetic acid (50 + 20 + 30 + 01, v/v)

Chamber saturation : —   *Migration distance :* 70 mm

Detection : UV (short) or iodine vapours

HRf : Spironolactone   25

         Furosemide   60

Comments : Chromatography on reversed-phase system gives better separation.

Reference : —

PROTOCOLS OF A THIN LAYER CHROMATOGRAM

Chromatogram No. 25

Formulation : Atenolol, Amlodipine besylate

Classification : Cardiac drugs

Dosage form : Tablets

Standard solution : Dissolve appropriate quantity of working standard of each drug substance in methanol for spotting.

Sample solution : Suspend powdered sample in methanol, sonicate for 5 min centrifuge and use the clear liquid for spotting.

Chromatographic conditions :

Test plate : TLC pre-coated plate, silica gel 60F$_{254}$

Format : 10 × 10 cm   *Thickness :* 250 μm

Volume spotted : 5 μl   *Separation technique :* Ascending

Mobile phase : 1. Toluene–acetone–methanol–ammonia (45 + 45 + 07 + 03, v/v)

                      2. Toluene–iso-propanol–ammonia (75 + 25 + 01, v/v)

Chamber saturation : 30 min   *Migration distance :* 70 mm

Detection : Atenolol UV (short); Amlodipine UV (long)

HRf : Atenolol   15

         Amlodipine besylate   65

Comments : —

Reference : —

PROTOCOLS OF A THIN LAYER CHROMATOGRAM

Chromatogram No. 26

Formulation : Enalapril maleate, Amlodipine besylate

Classification : Cardiac drugs

Dosage form : Tablets

Standard solution : See Chromatogram No. 25.

Sample solution : See Chromatogram No. 25.

Chromatographic conditions :

    Test plate : TLC pre-coated plate, silica gel 60F$_{254}$

    Format : 10 × 10 cm   *Thickness :* 250 μm

    Volume spotted : 10 μl   *Separation technique :* Ascending

    Mobile phase : Chloroform–methanol–glacial acetic acid (85 + 15 + 01, v/v)

    Chamber saturation : 10 min   *Migration distance :* 70 mm

    Detection : UV (short) or bromocresol solution (1%) in pH 3.0 phthalate buffer

    HRf :   Amlodipine besylate   35

           Enalapril maleate   65

Comments : —

Reference : —

Musculoskeletal Disorders

- **Analgesics and antipyretics**
- **Anti-inflammatory**
- **Muscle relaxants**

PROTOCOLS OF A THIN LAYER CHROMATOGRAM

Chromatogram No. 27

Formulation : Aspirin, Paracetamol, Caffeine citrate

Classification : Analgesic

Dosage form : Tablets

Standard solution : Dissolve appropriate quantity of each drug substance in methanol for spotting.

Sample solution : Suspend powdered sample in methanol, sonicate for 5 min, centrifuge and use the supernatant liquid for spotting.

Chromatographic conditions :

Test plate : TLC pre-coated plate, silica gel $60F_{254}$ or hand-made plate, silica gel GF_{254} (activate at 105°C for 30 min prior to use).

Format : 10 × 10 cm   *Thickness :* 250 µm

Volume spotted : 10 µl   *Separation technique :* Ascending

Mobile phase : 1. Toluene–methanol–ammonia (75 + 25 + 0.25, v/v)
2. n-hexane–ethyl acetate–glacial acetic acid (40 + 60 + 01, v/v)
3. Toluene–ethyl acetate–methanol–glacial acetic acid (50 + 40 + 10 + 01, v/v)
4. Ethyl acetate–glacial acetic acid (95 + 5, v/v)
5. Chloroform–glacial acetic acid–ethyl acetate (36 + 24 + 01, v/v)
6. Toluene–dioxane–glacial acetic acid (90 + 30 + 03, v/v)
7. Dichloromethane–iso-propanol–glacial acetic acid (21 + 03 + 0.2, v/v)

Chamber saturation : 30 min   *Migration distance :* 70 mm

Detection : UV (short) or iodine vapours

HRf :

	1	2	3	4	5	6	7
Aspirin	15	65	75	65	50	65	65
Paracetamol	55	25	60	50	50	48	10
Caffeine citrate	70	10	50	20	30	55	20

Comments : —

Reference : —

PROTOCOLS OF A THIN LAYER CHROMATOGRAM

Chromatogram No. 28

Formulation : Aspirin, Paracetamol, Caffeine citrate, Ascorbic acid
Classification : Analgesic
Dosage form : Tablets
Standard solution : See Chromatogram No. 27.
Sample solution : See Chromatogram No. 27.
Chromatographic conditions :

Test plate : Hand-made plate, silica gel GF$_{254}$ (activate at 105°C for 30 min prior to use).

Format : 10 × 20 cm   *Thickness :* 250 μm

Volume spotted : 10 μl   *Separation technique :* Ascending

Mobile phase :   1. Toluene–n-propanol–formic acid (75 + 25 + 01, v/v)

2. Dichloromethane–ethyl acetate–methanol (50 + 50 + 10, v/v)

Chamber saturation : 30 min   *Migration distance :* 150 mm

Detection : UV (short) or iodine vapours

HRf :

	1	2
Aspirin	30	30
Paracetamol	50	65
Caffeine citrate	35	45
Ascorbic acid	05	05

Comments : —
Reference : —

PROTOCOLS OF A THIN LAYER CHROMATOGRAM

Chromatogram No. 29

Formulation : Aspirin, Dipyridamole

Classification : Analgesic

Dosage form : Tablets

Standard solution : Dissolve working standard of each drug substance in methanol for spotting.

Sample solution : Suspend the powdered sample in methanol, sonicate for 5 min, centrifuge and use the supernatant solution for spotting.

Chromatographic conditions :

Test plate : TLC pre-coated plate, silica gel 60F$_{254}$

Format : 10 × 10 cm   *Thickness :* 250 μm

Volume spotted : 10 μl   *Separation technique :* Ascending

Mobile phase : 1. Chloroform–methanol–glacial acetic acid (95 + 05 + 0.4, v/v)

              2. Ethyl acetate–ethyl alcohol–13.5 M ammonia (15 + 03 + 03, v/v)

Chamber saturation : —   *Migration distance :* 70 mm

Detection : UV (short) or iodine vapours

HRf :	1	2
Aspirin	25	26
Dipyridamole	10	67

Comments : —

Reference : —

PROTOCOLS OF A THIN LAYER CHROMATOGRAM

Chromatogram No. 30

Formulation : Aspirin, Dipyridamole

Classification : Analgesic

Dosage form : Tablets

Standard solution : See Chromatogram No. 29.

Sample solution : See Chromatogram No. 29.

Chromatographic conditions :

Test plate : TLC pre-coated plate, silica gel 60F$_{254}$ impregnated with 5% silicone oil in petroleum ether (40-60)

Format : 10 × 10 cm   *Thickness :* 250 μm

Volume spotted : 10 μl   *Separation technique :* Ascending

Mobile phase : 0.5 M sodium chloride–methanol–acetonitrile–glacial acetic acid (50 + 20 + 30 + 01, v/v)

Chamber saturation : —   *Migration distance :* 70 mm

Detection : UV (short) or iodine vapours

HRf : Aspirin   80

  Dipyridamole   50

Comments : —

Reference : —

PROTOCOLS OF A THIN LAYER CHROMATOGRAM

Chromatogram No. 31

Formulation : Aspirin, Salicylamide, Salicylic acid

Classification : Analgesic

Dosage form : Tablets

Standard solution : Dissolve appropriate quantity of the working standard in methanol–n-hexane (1 : 1) for spotting.

Sample solution : Extract appropriate quantity of the powdered sample with methanol–n-hexane mixture (1 : 1) in ultrasonic water bath, centrifuge and use the clear solution for spotting.

Chromatographic conditions :

Test plate : TLC pre-coated plate, silica gel 60F$_{254}$

Format : 10 × 10 cm   *Thickness :* 250 μm

Volume spotted : 10 μl   *Separation technique :* Ascending

Mobile phase : Cyclohexane–chloroform–glacial acetic acid (60 + 05 + 05, v/v)

Chamber saturation : —   *Migration distance :* 70 mm

Detection : UV (short) or iodine vapours

HRf : Aspirin   20

      Salicylamide   07

      Salicylic acid   15

Comments : —

Reference : —

PROTOCOLS OF A THIN LAYER CHROMATOGRAM

Chromatogram No. 32

Formulation : Aspirin, Paracetamol, Codeine phosphate

Classification : Analgesic

Dosage form : Tablets, capsules

Standard solution : Dissolve appropriate quantity of each drug substance in methanol for spotting.

Sample solution : Extract the powdered sample with methanol by sonication, centrifuge and use the supernatant liquid for spotting.

Chromatographic conditions :

Test plate : Hand-made TLC plate, silica gel 60F$_{254}$ (activate at 105°C for 30 min prior to use).

Format : 10 × 20 cm   *Thickness :* 250 μm

Volume spotted : 10 μl   *Separation technique :* Ascending

Mobile phase :   1. Toluene–methanol–ammonia (75 + 25 + 0.25, v/v)

2. Butyl acetate–formic acid–chloroform (60 + 40 + 20, v/v)

3. Acetone–n-hexane–toluene–ammonia (30 + 30 + 10 + 0.25, v/v)

Chamber saturation : 30 min   *Migration distance :* 150 mm

Detection : UV (short) or iodine vapours

HRf :	1	2	3
Aspirin	15	85	05
Paracetamol	55	65	45
Codeine phosphate	40	20	15

Comments : —

Reference : —

PROTOCOLS OF A THIN LAYER CHROMATOGRAM

Chromatogram No. 33

Formulation : Aspirin, Paracetamol, Salicylamide

Classification : Analgesic

Dosage form : Tablets

Standard solution : See Chromatogram No. 32.

Sample solution : See Chromatogram No. 32.

Chromatographic conditions :

Test plate : Hand-made plate, silica gel GF$_{254}$ (activate at 105°C for 30 min prior to use).

Format : 10 × 20 cm   *Thickness :* 250 μm

Volume spotted : 10 μl   *Separation technique :* Ascending

Mobile phase : Toluene–methanol–ammonia (75 + 25 + 0.25, v/v)

Chamber saturation : 30 min   *Migration distance :* 120 mm

Detection : UV (short) or iodine vapours

HRf : Aspirin   15

Paracetamol   55

Salicylamide   70

Comments : —

Reference : —

PROTOCOLS OF A THIN LAYER CHROMATOGRAM

Chromatogram No. 34

Formulation : Aspirin, Paracetamol, Caffeine citrate, Chlorpheniramine maleate, Phenylephrine hydrochloride

Classification : Analgesic

Dosage form : Tablets, capsules

Standard solution : Prepare solution of each drug substance in methanol for spotting.

Sample solution : Suspend the powdered sample in methanol, sonicate for 10 min, decant, use the supernatant liquid for spotting.

Chromatographic conditions :

Test plate : Hand-made plate, silica gel GF$_{254}$

Format : 10 × 20 cm   *Thickness :* 250 μm

Volume spotted : 10 μl   *Separation technique :* Ascending

Mobile phase : 1. Toluene–methanol–ammonia (75 + 25 + 0.25, v/v)

                    2. Butyl acetate–formic acid–chloroform (60 + 40 + 20, v/v)

Chamber saturation : 30 min   *Migration distance :* 150 mm

Detection : UV (short) or iodine vapours

HRf :

	1	2
Aspirin	15	80
Paracetamol	55	65
Caffeine citrate	70	50
Chlorpheniramine maleate	30	30
Phenylephrine hydrochloride	08	20

Comments : —

Reference : —

PROTOCOLS OF A THIN LAYER CHROMATOGRAM

Chromatogram No. 35

Formulation : Aspirin, Caffeine citrate, Phenylephrine hydrochloride, Ascorbic acid
Classification : Analgesic
Dosage form : Tablets
Standard solution : See Chromatogram No. 34.
Sample solution : See Chromatogram No. 34.
Chromatographic conditions :

Test plate : Hand-made plate, silica gel GF$_{254}$ (activate prior to use, if required).

Format : 20 × 20 cm *Thickness* : 250 μm

Volume spotted : 10 μl *Separation technique* : Ascending

Mobile phase : 1. Toluene–methanol–ammonia (75 + 25 + 0.25, v/v)

2. Butyl acetate–formic acid–chloroform (60 + 40 + 20, v/v)

Chamber saturation : 30 min *Migration distance* : 150 mm

Detection : UV (short) or iodine vapours

HRf :	1	2
Aspirin	15	80
Caffeine citrate	70	50
Phenylephrine hydrochloride	08	20
Ascorbic acid	02	15

Comments : —
Reference : —

PROTOCOLS OF A THIN LAYER CHROMATOGRAM

Chromatogram No. 36

Formulation : Aspirin, Ethoheptazine citrate, Meprobamate

Classification : Analgesic

Dosage form : Tablets

Standard solution : Dissolve appropriate quantity of each working standard in methanol for application.

Sample solution : Suspend powdered sample in methanol, sonicate, centrifuge and use the supernatant for application.

Chromatographic conditions :

Test plate : Hand-made TLC plate, coated with silica gel GF$_{254}$ (activate at 105°C prior to use).

Format : 10 × 20 cm	*Thickness :* 250 μm
Volume spotted : 10 μl	*Separation technique :* Ascending

Mobile phase : Toluene–methanol–ammonia (75 + 25 + 0.25, v/v)

Chamber saturation : 15 min	*Migration distance :* 150 mm

Detection : Iodine vapours

HRf :

Aspirin	15
Ethoheptazine citrate	55
Meprobamate	70

Comments : —

Reference : —

PROTOCOLS OF A THIN LAYER CHROMATOGRAM

Chromatogram No. 37

Formulation : Paracetamol, Caffeine citrate, Analgin

Classification : Analgesic

Dosage form : Tablets

Standard solution : Dissolve appropriate quantity of working standard of each substance in methanol for application.

Sample solution : Suspend the powdered sample in methanol, slightly warm in water bath or sonicate for 15 min, centrifuge and use the supernatant for spotting.

Chromatographic conditions :

Test plate : Hand-made TLC plate, coated with silica gel GF_{254} (activate at 105°C prior to use).

Format : 10 × 20 cm *Thickness :* 250 μm

Volume spotted : 10 μl *Separation technique :* Ascending

Mobile phase : 1. Chloroform–methanol–toluene (90 + 10 + 10, v/v)

  2. Toluene–methanol–ammonia (75 + 25 + 0.25, v/v)

Chamber saturation : 15 min *Migration distance :* 150 mm

Detection : UV (short) or iodine vapours

HRf :

	1	2
Paracetamol	35	55
Caffeine citrate	65 - 70	
Analgin	06	20

Comments : —

Reference : —

PROTOCOLS OF A THIN LAYER CHROMATOGRAM

Chromatogram No. 38

Formulation : Paracetamol, Caffeine citrate, Analgin, Codeine phosphate
Classification : Analgesic
Dosage form : Tablets/capsules
Standard solution : See Chromatogram No. 37.
Sample solution : See Chromatogram No. 37.
Chromatographic conditions :

Test plate : Hand-made TLC plate, coated with silica gel GF$_{254}$ (activate at 105°C prior to use).

Format : 10 × 20 cm   *Thickness :* 250 μm

Volume spotted : 10 μl   *Separation technique :* Ascending

Mobile phase :   1. Chloroform–methanol–toluene (85 + 15 + 10, v/v)
               2. Toluene–methanol–ammonia (75 + 25 + 0.25, v/v)
               3. Toluene–ethyl acetate–ammonia (50 + 50 + 0.2, v/v)
               4. Chloroform–cyclohexane–acetone–diethylamine (60 + 20 + 10 + 10, v/v)

Chamber saturation : 30 min   *Migration distance :* 150 mm

Detection : UV (short) or iodine vapours

HRƒ :

	1	2	3	4
Paracetamol	40	55	45	15
Caffeine citrate	65	70	20	45
Analgin	07	20	30	10
Codeine phosphate	55	40	08	35

Comments : —
Reference : —

PROTOCOLS OF A THIN LAYER CHROMATOGRAM

Chromatogram No. 39

Formulation : Paracetamol, Analgin, Chloroquine phosphate

Classification : Analgesic

Dosage form : Tablets

Standard solution : Dissolve appropriate quantity of each working standard in 2 ml of water and further dilute with methanol for application.

Sample solution : Suspend the powdered sample in 2 ml of water, add methanol, sonicate, filter and use the filtrate for application.

Chromatographic conditions :

Test plate : Hand-made TLC plate, coated with silica gel GF$_{254}$ (activate at 105°C for 30 min prior to use).

Format : 10 × 20 cm   *Thickness :* 250 μm

Volume spotted : 10 μl   *Separation technique :* Ascending

Mobile phase : Toluene–methanol–ammonia (75 + 25 + 0.25, v/v)

Chamber saturation : 30 min   *Migration distance :* 150 mm

Detection : UV (short) or iodine vapours

HRf :   Paracetamol   55

       Analgin   20

       Chloroquine phosphate   10

Comments : —

Reference : —

PROTOCOLS OF A THIN LAYER CHROMATOGRAM

Chromatogram No. 40

Formulation : Paracetamol, Caffeine citrate, Propyphenazone

Classification : Analgesic

Dosage form : Tablets

Standard solution : Dissolve working standard of each drug substance in methanol for application.

Sample solution : Suspend appropriate quantity of powdered sample in methanol, sonicate, filter and use the filtrate.

Chromatographic conditions :

Test plate : Hand-made TLC plate, coated with silica gel GF$_{254}$.

Format : 10 × 10 cm   *Thickness :* 250 μm

Volume spotted : 5 μl   *Separation technique :* Ascending

Mobile phase :   1. n-hexane–ethyl acetate–glacial acetic acid (50 + 50 + 01, v/v)

2. Chloroform–dioxane (75 + 25, v/v)

3. Butyl acetate–formic acid–chloroform (60 + 40 + 20, v/v)

4. Chloroform–methanol (90 + 10, v/v)

Chamber saturation : 30 min   *Migration distance :* 70 mm

Detection : UV (short) or iodine vapours

HRf :	1	2	3	4
Paracetamol	25	25	65	75
Caffeine citrate	10	45	50	40
Propyphenazone	70	80	40	35

Comments : —

Reference : —

PROTOCOLS OF A THIN LAYER CHROMATOGRAM

Chromatogram No. 41

Formulation : Paracetamol, Caffeine citrate, Propoxyphene

Classification : Analgesic

Dosage form : Tablets

Standard solution : See Chromatogram No. 40.

Sample solution : See Chromatogram No. 40.

Chromatographic conditions :

Test plate : Pre-coated TLC plate, silica gel 60GF$_{254}$ impregnated with 5% silicone oil in petroleum ether (40-60).

Format : 10 × 10 cm   *Thickness :* 250 μm

Volume spotted : 5 μl   *Separation technique :* Ascending

Mobile phase : 0.5 M sodium chloride–methanol–glacial acetic acid (120 + 80 + 0.1, v/v)

Chamber saturation : 30 min   *Migration distance :* 70 mm

Detection : UV (short) or iodine vapours

HRf :   Paracetamol   80

        Caffeine citrate   55

        Propyphenazone   20

Comments : —

Reference : —

PROTOCOLS OF A THIN LAYER CHROMATOGRAM

Chromatogram No. 42

Formulation : Paracetamol, Caffeine citrate, Phenyldimethyl isopropylpyrazolone, Diethyl-dioxo-tetrahydropyriline

Classification : Analgesic

Dosage form : Tablets/capsules

Standard solution : Dissolve working standard of each drug substance in mixture of chloroform–methanol (1 + 1) for application.

Sample solution : Suspend powdered sample in chloroform–methanol (1 + 1) mixture, slightly warm, centrifuge and use the supernatant.

Chromatographic conditions :

Test plate : Hand-made TLC plate, coated with silica gel GF$_{254}$ (activate at 105°C prior to use).

Format : 10 × 20 cm   *Thickness :* 250 μm

Volume spotted : 10 μl   *Separation technique :* Ascending

Mobile phase : Chloroform–ethyl acetate (1 + 1, v/v)

Chamber saturation : 30 min   *Migration distance :* 150 mm

Detection : UV (short) or iodine vapours

HRf : Paracetamol   40
         Caffeine citrate   25
         Phenyldimethyl isopropylpyrazolone   75
         Diethyl-dioxo-tetrahydropyriline   60

Comments : —

Reference : —

PROTOCOLS OF A THIN LAYER CHROMATOGRAM

Chromatogram No. 43

Formulation : Paracetamol, Caffeine citrate, Ascorbic acid

Classification : Analgesic

Dosage form : Tablets

Standard solution : Dissolve working standard of each drug substance in 80% methanol for application.

Sample solution : Powdered sample is suspended in 80% methanol, sonicate for 5-10 min, centrifuge and use the supernatant.

Chromatographic conditions :

Test plate : Hand-made TLC plate, coated with silica gel GF_{254} (activate at 105°C for 30 min prior to use).

Format : 10 × 20 cm   *Thickness :* 250 μm

Volume spotted : 10 μl   *Separation technique :* Ascending

Mobile phase :   1. Dichloromethane–ethyl acetate–methanol (50 + 50 + 10, v/v)
                      2. Toluene–methanol–ammonia (75 + 25 + 0.25, v/v)

Chamber saturation : 30 min   *Migration distance :* 150 mm

Detection : UV (short) or iodine vapours

HRf :	1	2
Paracetamol	55	50
Caffeine citrate	45	70
Ascorbic acid	05	02

Comments : —

Reference : —

PROTOCOLS OF A THIN LAYER CHROMATOGRAM

Chromatogram No. 44

Formulation : Paracetamol, Caffeine citrate, Ascorbic acid
Classification : Analgesic
Dosage form : Tablets
Standard solution : See Chromatogram No. 43.
Sample solution : See Chromatogram No. 43.
Chromatographic conditions :

Test plate : Hand-made TLC plate, coated with silica gel GF_{254} impregnated with 5% silicone oil in petroleum ether (40-60).

Format : 10 × 20 cm	*Thickness :* 250 µm
Volume spotted : 10 µl	*Separation technique :* Ascending

Mobile phase : Methanol–water–acetic acid (47 + 50 + 03, v/v)

Chamber saturation :	*Migration distance :* 100 mm

Detection : UV (short) or iodine vapours

HRf :	Paracetamol	60
	Caffeine citrate	25
	Ascorbic acid	85

Comments : —
Reference : —

PROTOCOLS OF A THIN LAYER CHROMATOGRAM

Chromatogram No. 45

Formulation : Paracetamol, Caffeine citrate, Phenylephrine hydrochloride, Chlorpheniramine maleate

Classification : Analgesic

Dosage form : Tablets/capsules

Standard solution : Dissolve working standard of each drug substance in methanol for application.

Sample solution : Suspend powdered sample in 2 ml of water, shake, add methanol, sonicate, centrifuge and use the supernatant for spotting.

Chromatographic conditions :

Test plate : Hand-made TLC plate, coated with silica gel GF$_{254}$ (activate at 105°C prior to use).

Format : 10 × 20 cm   *Thickness :* 250 μm

Volume spotted : 10 μl   *Separation technique :* Ascending

Mobile phase :   1. Toluene–methanol–ammonia (75 + 25 + 0.25, v/v)

                            2. Butyl acetate–formic acid–chloroform (60 + 40 + 20, v/v)

Chamber saturation : 30 min   *Migration distance :* 150 mm

Detection : UV (short) or iodine vapours

HRf :	1	2
Paracetamol	50	50
Caffeine citrate	70	65
Phenylephrine hydrochloride	08	20
Chlorpheniramine maleate	30	30

Comments : —

Reference : —

PROTOCOLS OF A THIN LAYER CHROMATOGRAM

Chromatogram No. 46

Formulation : Paracetamol, Caffeine citrate, Ascorbic acid, Phenylephrine hydro-chloride

Classification : Analgesic

Dosage form : Tablets

Standard solution : See Chromatogram No. 43.

Sample solution : See Chromatogram No. 43.

Chromatographic conditions :

Test plate : Pre-coated TLC plate, silica gel 60F$_{254}$

Format : 10 × 10 cm   Thickness : 250 μm

Volume spotted : 5 μl   Separation technique : Ascending

Mobile phase : Methylene chloride–ethyl acetate–methanol–formic acid (35 + 20 + 40 + 05, v/v)

Chamber saturation : 15 min   Migration distance : 70 mm

Detection : UV (short) or iodine vapours

HRf :   Paracetamol   85
        Caffeine citrate   65
        Ascorbic acid   50
        Phenylephrine hydrochloride   22

Comments : —

Reference : —

PROTOCOLS OF A THIN LAYER CHROMATOGRAM

Chromatogram No. 47

Formulation : Paracetamol, Phenylephrine hydrochloride, Triprolidine hydrochloride

Classification : Analgesic

Dosage form : Tablets

Standard solution : Dissolve working standard of each drug substance in 80% aqueous methanol for spotting.

Sample solution : Suspend the powdered sample in methanol, sonicate for 10 min, centrifuge and use the supernatant for spotting.

Chromatographic conditions :

Test plate : Pre-coated TLC plate, silica gel 60F$_{254}$

Format : 10 × 10 cm   *Thickness :* 250 μm

Volume spotted : 5 μl   *Separation technique :* Ascending

Mobile phase : Toluene–acetone–iso-propanol–ammonia (60 + 30 + 20 + 03, v/v)

Chamber saturation : 30 min   *Migration distance :* 70 mm

Detection : Visible (spray with 0.2% ninhydrin solution, heat in the oven (105°C) for 30 min

HRf : Paracetamol   58

Phenylephrine hydrochloride   49

Triprolidine hydrochloride   75

Diphenhydramine hydrochloride (IS)   40

Comments : —

Reference : J.L. Chawla, R.A. Sodhi and R.T. Sane. Indian Drugs, 34 (6), 339-340, 1997.

PROTOCOLS OF A THIN LAYER CHROMATOGRAM

Chromatogram No. 48

Formulation : Paracetamol, Pentazocine hydrochloride

Classification : Analgesic

Dosage form : Tablets

Standard solution : Working standard of each drug substance is dissolved in methanol for spotting.

Sample solution : Extract powdered sample with methanol by shaking for 5-10 min, filter and use the filtrate for spotting.

Chromatographic conditions :

Test plate : Hand-made TLC plate, coated with silica gel GF$_{254}$ (activate at 105°C for 30 min prior to use).

Format : 10 × 20 cm   *Thickness :* 250 µm

Volume spotted : 5 µl   *Separation technique :* Ascending

Mobile phase : 1. Toluene–acetone–ammonia (60 + 40 + 01, v/v)

                          2. Toluene–ethyl acetate–acetone–ammonia (50 + 50 + 05 + 0.2, v/v)

Chamber saturation : 30 min   *Migration distance :* 150 mm

Detection : UV (short) or iodine vapours

HRf :

	1	2
Paracetamol	30	45
Pentazocine hydrochloride	50	10

Comments : —

Reference : —

PROTOCOLS OF A THIN LAYER CHROMATOGRAM

Chromatogram No. 49

Formulation : **Paracetamol, Ibuprofen**

Classification : Analgesic

Dosage form : Tablets

Standard solution : Appropriate quantity of each working standard is taken up in methanol for spotting.

Sample solution : Suspend the powdered sample in methanol, sonicate, centrifuge and use the supernatant for spotting.

Chromatographic conditions :

Test plate : Hand-made TLC plate, coated with silica gel GF$_{254}$ (activate at 105°C for 30 min prior to use).

Format : 10 × 20 cm   *Thickness :* 250 μm

Volume spotted : 10 μl   *Separation technique :* Ascending

Mobile phase :   1. n-hexane–ethyl acetate–acetic acid (150 + 50 + 10, v/v)

2. n-hexane–ethyl acetate–acetic acid (90 + 25 + 10, v/v)

3. Butyl acetate–formic acid–chloroform (60 + 40 + 20, v/v)

Chamber saturation : 30 min   *Migration distance :* 150 mm

Detection : UV (short) or iodine vapours or spray with 1% w/v solution of potassium permanganate in dilute sulphuric acid

HRf :

	1	2	3
Paracetamol	20	10	60
Ibuprofen	70	80	75

Comments : —

Reference : —

PROTOCOLS OF A THIN LAYER CHROMATOGRAM

Chromatogram No. 50

Formulation : Paracetamol, Metoclopramide hydrochloride

Classification : Analgesic

Dosage form : Tablets

Standard solution : Prepare solution of each drug substance in methanol for spotting.

Sample solution : Extract the powdered sample with methanol by shaking, filter and use the filtrate for spotting.

Chromatographic conditions :

Test plate : Hand-made TLC plate, coated with silica gel GF$_{254}$ (activate at 105°C for 30 min prior to use).

Format : 10 × 20 cm   *Thickness :* 250 µm

Volume spotted : 10 µl   *Separation technique :* Ascending

Mobile phase :   1. Toluene–methanol–ammonia (75 + 25 + 0.25, v/v)

  2. Toluene–ethyl acetate–acetone–ammonia (50 + 50 + 05 + 0.2, v/v)

  3. Ethyl acetate–acetone–ammonia (60 + 40 + 01, v/v)

Chamber saturation : 30 min   *Migration distance :* 150 mm

Detection : UV (short) or iodine vapours

HRf :	1	2	3
Paracetamol	55	45	65
Metoclopramide hydrochloride	40	10	25

Comments : —

Reference : —

PROTOCOLS OF A THIN LAYER CHROMATOGRAM

Chromatogram No. 51

Formulation : Paracetamol, Ibuprofen, Dextropropoxyphene hydrochloride
Classification : Analgesic
Dosage form : Tablets
Standard solution : Prepare solution of working standard of each drug substance in methanol for spotting.
Sample solution : Suspend the powdered sample in methanol, sonicate for 5 min, centrifuge and use the supernatant for spotting.
Chromatographic conditions :

Test plate : Hand-made TLC plate, coated with silica gel GF_{254} (activate at 105°C for 30 min prior to use).

Format : 10 × 20 cm *Thickness :* 250 μm

Volume spotted : 10 μl *Separation technique :* Ascending

Mobile phase : 1. Toluene–acetone–glacial acetic acid (70 + 30 + 05, v/v)
 2. Toluene–methanol–ammonia (75 + 25 + 0.25, v/v)

Chamber saturation : 30 min *Migration distance :* 150 mm

Detection : Iodine vapours

HRf :	1	2
Paracetamol	10	55
Ibuprofen	45	40
Dextropropoxyphene hydrochloride	60	85

Comments : —
Reference : —

PROTOCOLS OF A THIN LAYER CHROMATOGRAM

Chromatogram No. 52

Formulation : Paracetamol, Codeine phosphate

Classification : Analgesic

Dosage form : Tablets

Standard solution : See Chromatogram No. 38.

Sample solution : See Chromatogram No. 38.

Chromatographic conditions :

Test plate : Pre-coated TLC plate, silica gel $60F_{254}$

Format : 10 × 10 cm   Thickness : 200 μm

Volume spotted : 5 μl   Separation technique : Ascending

Mobile phase :   1. Toluene–n-propanol–ammonia (60 + 40 + 04, v/v)

               2. Chloroform–methanol–toluene (85 + 15 + 10, v/v)

Chamber saturation : —   Migration distance : 70 mm

Detection : UV (short) or iodine vapours or spray with Dragendorff's reagent

HRf :

	1	2
Paracetamol	70	55
Codeine phosphate	45	40

Comments : —

Reference : —

PROTOCOLS OF A THIN LAYER CHROMATOGRAM

Chromatogram No. 53

Formulation : Paracetamol, Codeine phosphate

Classification : Analgesic

Dosage form : Tablets

Standard solution : See Chromatogram No. 38.

Sample solution : See Chromatogram No. 38.

Chromatographic conditions :

Test plate : Reversed-phase HPTLC pre-coated plate, silica gel 60RP-18F$_{254s}$

Format : 5 × 10 cm   *Thickness :* 100 μm

Volume spotted : 5 μl   *Separation technique :* Ascending

Mobile phase : Methanol–0.5 M phosphate buffer (pH 8.5) (40 + 60, v/v)

Chamber saturation : —   *Migration distance :* 50 mm

Detection : UV (short) or iodine vapours

HRf : Paracetamol   60

       Codeine phosphate   15

Comments : —

Reference : —

PROTOCOLS OF A THIN LAYER CHROMATOGRAM

Chromatogram No. 54

Formulation : Paracetamol, Chlormezanone

Classification : Analgesic and muscle relaxants

Dosage form : Tablets

Standard solution : Prepare solution of working standard of each drug substance in methanol for spotting.

Sample solution : Suspend appropriate quantity of the powdered sample in methanol, sonicate, centrifuge and use the supernatant for spotting.

Chromatographic conditions :

Test plate : Pre-coated TLC plate, silica gel 60F$_{254}$

Format : 10 × 10 cm   *Thickness :* 250 μm

Volume spotted : 5 μl   *Separation technique :* Ascending

Mobile phase :   1. Toluene–methanol–ammonia (75 + 25 + 0.25, v/v)

                            2. n-hexane–ethyl acetate–glacial acetic acid (70 + 50 + 10, v/v)

Chamber saturation : 30 min   *Migration distance :* 70 mm

Detection : UV (short) or iodine vapours

HRf :

	1	2
Paracetamol	55	20
Chlormezanone	80	30

Comments : —

Reference : —

PROTOCOLS OF A THIN LAYER CHROMATOGRAM

Chromatogram No. 55

Formulation : Paracetamol, Chlormezanone

Classification : Analgesic

Dosage form : Tablets

Standard solution : See Chromatogram No. 54.

Sample solution : See Chromatogram No. 54.

Chromatographic conditions :

Test plate : Pre-coated TLC plate, silica gel 60F$_{254}$, impregnated with 5% silicone oil in petroleum ether (40-60).

Format : 10 × 10 cm   *Thickness :* 250 μm

Volume spotted : 5 μl   *Separation technique :* Ascending

Mobile phase : 0.5 M sodium chloride–methanol–glacial acetic acid (120 + 80 + 0.1, v/v)

Chamber saturation : 30 min   *Migration distance :* 70 mm

Detection : UV (short) or iodine vapours

HRf :   Paracetamol   70

       Chlormezanone   35

Comments : See reversal of retention order (Rf) as compared to normal-phase chromatography.

Reference : —

PROTOCOLS OF A THIN LAYER CHROMATOGRAM

Chromatogram No. 56

Formulation : Paracetamol, Analgin, Diazepam, Chlorpheniramine maleate

Classification : Analgesic

Dosage form : Tablets

Standard solution : Prepare the solution of each substance in methanol for application.

Sample solution : Extract the powdered sample with methanol in ultrasonic water-bath (5 min), filter and use the filtrate for spotting.

Chromatographic conditions :

Test plate : Hand-made TLC plate, coated with silica gel GF_{254} (activate at 105°C prior to use).

Format : 10 × 20 cm   *Thickness :* 250 μm

Volume spotted : 10 μl   *Separation technique :* Ascending

Mobile phase : 1. Toluene–methanol–ammonia (75 + 25 + 0.25, v/v)

                          2. Butyl acetate–formic acid–chloroform (60 + 40 + 20, v/v)

Chamber saturation : 30 min   *Migration distance :* 150 mm

Detection : Iodine vapours

HRf :

	1	2
Paracetamol	55	45
Analgin	20	30
Diazepam	75	25
Chlorpheniramine maleate	30	10

Comments : —

Reference : —

PROTOCOLS OF A THIN LAYER CHROMATOGRAM

Chromatogram No. 57

Formulation : Paracetamol, Dicyclomine hydrochloride, Diazepam, Dextro-propoxyphene hydrochloride

Classification : Analgesic

Dosage form : Tablets/capsules

Standard solution : Prepare solution of each drug substance separately in methanol for spotting.

Sample solution : Suspend the powdered sample in methanol, sonicate, centrifuge and use the supernatant for spotting.

Chromatographic conditions :

Test plate : Hand-made TLC plate, coated with silica gel GF$_{254}$

Format : 10 × 20 cm   *Thickness :* 250 μm

Volume spotted : 10 μl   *Separation technique :* Ascending

Mobile phase :   1. Toluene–acetone–ammonia (70 + 30 + 0.5, v/v)

    2. Ethyl acetate–chloroform–methanol–water–ammonia (75 + 15 + 05 + 03 + 02, v/v)

Chamber saturation : 30 min   *Migration distance :* 150 mm

Detection : UV (short) or iodine vapours

HRƒ :

	1	2
Paracetamol	65	20
Dicyclomine hydrochloride	20	60
Diazepam	80	85
Dextropropoxyphene hydrochloride	35	70

Comments : —

Reference : —

PROTOCOLS OF A THIN LAYER CHROMATOGRAM

Chromatogram No. 58

Formulation : Paracetamol, Dicyclomine hydrochloride, Mefenamic acid

Classification : Analgesic

Dosage form : Tablets

Standard solution : See Chromatogram No. 57.

Sample solution : See Chromatogram No. 57.

Chromatographic conditions :

Test plate : Hand-made TLC plate, coated with silica gel GF_{254}

Format : 10×20 cm   *Thickness :* 250 μm

Volume spotted : 10 μl   *Separation technique :* Ascending

Mobile phase : 1. Toluene–methanol–ammonia (75 + 25 + 0.25, v/v)

              2. Toluene–acetone–methanol–ammonia (70 + 20 + 10 + 0.2, v/v)

              3. Toluene–acetone–ammonia (70 + 30 + 0.5, v/v)

              4. n-hexane–ethyl acetate–glacial acetic acid (150 + 50 + 10, v/v)

              5. Butyl acetate–formic acid–chloroform (60 + 40 + 20, v/v)

Chamber saturation : 30 min   *Migration distance :* 150 mm

Detection : UV (short) or iodine vapours

HRf :

	1	2	3	4	5
Paracetamol	55	—	20	20	60
Dicyclomine hydrochloride	75	70	65	—	—
Mefenamic acid	40	20	—	80	85

Comments : —

Reference : —

PROTOCOLS OF A THIN LAYER CHROMATOGRAM

Chromatogram No. 59

Formulation : Paracetamol, Caffeine citrate, Dextropropoxyphene hydrochloride

Classification : Analgesic

Dosage form : Tablets/capsules

Standard solution : See Chromatogram No. 57.

Sample solution : See Chromatogram No. 57.

Chromatographic conditions :

Test plate : Hand-made TLC plate, coated with silica gel GF$_{254}$ (activate at 105°C prior to use).

Format : 10 × 20 cm   *Thickness :* 250 μm

Volume spotted : 10 μl   *Separation technique :* Ascending

Mobile phase :   1. Toluene–methanol–ammonia (75 + 25 + 0.25, v/v)

                          2. Butyl acetate–formic acid–chloroform (60 + 40 + 20, v/v)

Chamber saturation : 30 min   *Migration distance :* 150 mm

Detection : UV (short) or iodine vapours

HRf :	1	2
Paracetamol	55	65
Caffeine citrate	70	50
Dextropropoxyphene hydrochloride	85	80

Comments : —

Reference : —

PROTOCOLS OF A THIN LAYER CHROMATOGRAM

Chromatogram No. 60

Formulation : Paracetamol, Diclofenac sodium

Classification : Analgesic

Dosage form : Tablets

Standard solution : Dissolve working standard of both the substances in methanol (80%) for spotting.

Sample solution : Prepare sample solution by shaking appropriate quantity of powdered sample with methanol, centrifuge and use supernatant for spotting.

Chromatographic conditions :

Test plate : Pre-coated TLC plate, silica gel 60F$_{254}$

Format : 10 × 10 cm   *Thickness :* 250 μm

Volume spotted : 5 μl   *Separation technique :* Ascending

Mobile phase : 1. n-hexane–ethyl acetate–glacial acetic acid (90 + 25 + 10, v/v)
            2. Chloroform–methanol–ammonia (100 + 50 + 01, v/v)

Chamber saturation : 30 min   *Migration distance :* 70 mm

Detection : UV (short) or spray with ferric chloride solution

HRf :

	1	2
Paracetamol	75	10
Diclofenac sodium	35	70

Comments : —

Reference : —

PROTOCOLS OF A THIN LAYER CHROMATOGRAM

Formulation : **Paracetamol, Diclofenac sodium**

Classification : Analgesic

Dosage form : Tablets

Standard solution : See Chromatogram No. 60.

Sample solution : See Chromatogram No. 60.

Chromatographic conditions :

Test plate : Pre-coated TLC plate, silica gel 60F$_{254}$, impregnated with 5% silicone oil in petroleum ether (40-60).

Format : 10 × 10 cm   *Thickness* : 250 μm

Volume spotted : 5 μl   *Separation technique* : Ascending

Mobile phase : 0.5 M sodium chloride–methanol–glacial acetic acid (120 + 80 + 0.1, v/v)

Chamber saturation : 30 min   *Migration distance* : 70 mm

Detection : UV (short) or spray with 1% solution of ferric chloride

HRf : Paracetamol   75

      Diclofenac sodium   40

Comments : —

Reference : —

PROTOCOLS OF A THIN LAYER CHROMATOGRAM

Chromatogram No. 62

Formulation : Paracetamol, Diclofenac sodium, Chlorzoxazone
Classification : Analgesic and muscle relaxant
Dosage form : Tablets
Standard solution : See Chromatogram No. 60.
Sample solution : See Chromatogram No. 60.
Chromatographic conditions :

Test plate : Pre-coated TLC plate, silica gel $60F_{254}$

Format : 10×10 cm   *Thickness :* 250 µm

Volume spotted : 5 µl   *Separation technique :* Ascending

Mobile phase :   1. Toluene–ethyl acetate–glacial acetic acid (60 + 40 + 0.2, v/v)
                   2. Toluene–acetone (70 + 30, v/v)

Chamber saturation : 15 min   *Migration distance :* 70 mm

Detection : UV (short) or iodine vapours

HRf :

	1	2
Paracetamol	15	25
Diclofenac sodium	30	55
Chlorzoxazone	65	70

Comments : —
Reference : —

PROTOCOLS OF A THIN LAYER CHROMATOGRAM

Chromatogram No. 63

Formulation : Paracetamol, Chlorzoxazone

Classification : Analgesic and muscle relaxant

Dosage form : Tablets

Standard solution : See Chromatogram No. 60.

Sample solution : See Chromatogram No. 60.

Chromatographic conditions :

Test plate : Pre-coated TLC plate, silica gel 60F$_{254}$, impregnated with 5% silicone oil in petroleum ether (40-60).

Format : 5 × 10 cm   *Thickness :* 250 µm

Volume spotted : 5 µl   *Separation technique :* Ascending

Mobile phase : 0.5 M sodium chloride–methanol–glacial acetic acid (120 + 80 + 0.1, v/v)

Chamber saturation : 30 min   *Migration distance :* 70 mm

Detection : Iodine vapours

HRf : Paracetamol   65

         Chlorzoxazone   20

Comments : See reversal of retention time as compared to normal-phase chromatography (Chromatogram No. 62).

Reference : —

PROTOCOLS OF A THIN LAYER CHROMATOGRAM

Chromatogram No. 64

Formulation : Paracetamol, Ibuprofen, Chlorzoxazone

Classification : Analgesic and muscle relaxant

Dosage form : Tablets

Standard solution : Dissolve appropriate quantity of each working standard in methanol for spotting.

Sample solution : Suspend powdered sample in methanol, shake in vortex mixture for 5 min, filter and use the filtrate for spotting.

Chromatographic conditions :

Test plate : Pre-coated TLC plate, silica gel 60F$_{254}$

Format : 10 × 10 cm   *Thickness :* 250 µm

Volume spotted : 5 µl   *Separation technique :* Ascending

Mobile phase : 1. Toluene–ethyl acetate–glacial acetic acid (60 + 30 + 05, v/v)

                 2. Chloroform–toluene–dioxane (70 + 20 + 20, v/v)

Chamber saturation : 30 min   *Migration distance :* 70 mm

Detection : Iodine vapours

HRf :	1	2
Paracetamol	30	25
Ibuprofen	80	85
Chlorzoxazone	70	70

Comments : —

Reference : —

PROTOCOLS OF A THIN LAYER CHROMATOGRAM

Formulation : Paracetamol, Ketoprofen, Chlorzoxazone

Classification : Analgesic and muscle relaxant

Dosage form : Tablets

Standard solution : See Chromatogram No. 64.

Sample solution : See Chromatogram No. 64.

Chromatographic conditions :

Test plate : Pre-coated TLC plate, silica gel 60F$_{254}$

Format : 10 × 10 cm　　　　　　*Thickness :* 250 µm

Volume spotted : 5 µl　　　　　*Separation technique :* Ascending

Mobile phase : Toluene–ethyl acetate–glacial acetic acid (60 + 40 + 02, v/v)

Chamber saturation : 30 min　　*Migration distance :* 70 mm

Detection : Iodine vapours

HRf :　Paracetamol　　　　　　15

　　　　Ketoprofen　　　　　　30

　　　　Chlorzoxazone　　　　　65

Comments : —

Reference : —

PROTOCOLS OF A THIN LAYER CHROMATOGRAM

Chromatogram No. 66

Formulation : **Paracetamol, Dicyclomine hydrochloride, Chlordiazepoxide**

Classification : Analgesic

Dosage form : Tablets

Standard solution : Prepare solution of working standard of each drug substance in methanol for spotting.

Sample solution : Suspend powdered sample in methanol, shake, filter and use the filtrate for spotting.

Chromatographic conditions :

Test plate : Hand-made TLC plate, coated with silica gel GF$_{254}$ (activate at 105°C prior to use).

Format : 10 × 20 cm   *Thickness :* 250 µm

Volume spotted : 10 µl   *Separation technique :* Ascending

Mobile phase :   1. Toluene–methanol–ammonia (75 + 25 + 0.25, v/v)

2. Toluene–ethyl acetate–acetone–ammonia (50 + 50 + 05 + 0.2, v/v)

Chamber saturation : 30 min   *Migration distance :* 150 mm

Detection : UV (short) or iodine vapours

HRf :

	1	2
Paracetamol	55	45
Dicyclomine hydrochloride	80	80
Chlordiazepoxide	70	20

Comments : —

Reference : —

PROTOCOLS OF A THIN LAYER CHROMATOGRAM

Formulation : Paracetamol, Methocarbamol

Classification : Analgesic and muscle relaxant

Dosage form : Tablets

Standard solution : Appropriate quantity of each working standard is dissolved in methanol for spotting.

Sample solution : Suspend powdered sample in methanol, sonicate, filter and use the filtrate for spotting.

Chromatographic conditions :

Test plate : Hand-made TLC plate, coated with silica gel GF$_{254}$ (may be activated at 105°C prior to use).

Format : 10 × 20 cm   *Thickness :* 250 µm

Volume spotted : 10 µl   *Separation technique :* Ascending

Mobile phase : Chloroform–methanol–glacial acetic acid (95 + 05 + 02, v/v)

Chamber saturation : 30 min   *Migration distance :* 150 mm

Detection : UV (short) or iodine vapours

HRf : Paracetamol   20

         Methocarbamol   40

Comments : —

Reference : —

PROTOCOLS OF A THIN LAYER CHROMATOGRAM

Chromatogram No. 68

Formulation : Paracetamol, Methocarbamol

Classification : Analgesic and muscle relaxant

Dosage form : Tablets

Standard solution : See Chromatogram No. 67.

Sample solution : See Chromatogram No. 67.

Chromatographic conditions :

Test plate : Hand-made TLC plate, coated with silica gel GF_{254}, impregnated with 5% silicone oil in petroleum ether (40-60).

Format : 10 × 20 cm   *Thickness :* 250 µm

Volume spotted : 10 µl   *Separation technique :* Ascending

Mobile phase : 0.5 M sodium chloride–methanol–glacial acetic acid (120 + 80 + 0.1, v/v)

Chamber saturation : 30 min   *Migration distance :* 150 mm

Detection : UV (short) or iodine vapours

HRf :   Paracetamol   70

        Methocarbamol   40

Comments : See reversal of retention order as compared to normal-phase chromatography.

Reference : —

PROTOCOLS OF A THIN LAYER CHROMATOGRAM

Chromatogram No. 69

Formulation : Paracetamol, Ketoprofen

Classification : Analgesic

Dosage form : Tablets

Standard solution : Dissolve both the substances separately in methanol for spotting.

Sample solution : Extract the sample with methanol by sonicating, filter and use the filtrate.

Chromatographic conditions :

Test plate : Pre-coated TLC plate, silica gel 60F$_{254}$

Format : 10 × 10 cm   *Thickness :* 250 µm

Volume spotted : 5 µl   *Separation technique :* Ascending

Mobile phase : Chloroform–acetone–methanol–glacial acetic acid (90 + 05 + 05 + 0.2, v/v)

Chamber saturation : 30 min   *Migration distance :* 70 mm

Detection : UV (short) or iodine vapours

HRf : Paracetamol   20
         Ketoprofen   35

Comments : —

Reference : —

PROTOCOLS OF A THIN LAYER CHROMATOGRAM

Chromatogram No. 70

Formulation : Paracetamol, Ketoprofen
Classification : Analgesic
Dosage form : Tablets
Standard solution : See Chromatogram No. 69.
Sample solution : See Chromatogram No. 69.
Chromatographic conditions :

Test plate : Reversed-phase HPTLC plate, silica gel 60RP-18F$_{254s}$

Format : 5 × 10 cm   *Thickness :* 100 μm

Volume spotted : 5 μl   *Separation technique :* Ascending

Mobile phase : 0.5 M sodium chloride–methanol–glacial acetic acid (120 + 80 + 0.1, v/v)

Chamber saturation : —   *Migration distance :* 50 mm

Detection : UV (short) or iodine vapours

HRf : Paracetamol   60
         Ketoprofen   25

Comments : See reversal of retention order as compared to normal-phase chromatography.
Reference : —

PROTOCOLS OF A THIN LAYER CHROMATOGRAM

Chromatogram No. 71

Formulation : Paracetamol, Naproxen
Classification : Analgesic
Dosage form : Tablets
Standard solution : See Chromatogram No. 69.
Sample solution : See Chromatogram No. 69.
Chromatographic conditions :

Test plate : Hand-made TLC plate, coated with silica gel GF_{254} (activate at 105°C prior to use).

Format : 10 × 10 cm   *Thickness :* 250 μm

Volume spotted : 10 μl   *Separation technique :* Ascending

Mobile phase : Chloroform–methanol–ammonia (90 + 10 + 0.6, v/v)

Chamber saturation : 30 min   *Migration distance :* 70 mm

Detection : UV (short) or iodine vapours

HRf : Paracetamol   35
          Naproxen   15

Comments : —
Reference : —

PROTOCOLS OF A THIN LAYER CHROMATOGRAM

Chromatogram No. 72

Formulation : Paracetamol, Oxyphenbutazone

Classification : Analgesic and anti-inflammatory

Dosage form : Tablets

Standard solution : Dissolve appropriate quantity of each working standard in methanol for spotting.

Sample solution : Suspend powdered sample in methanol, sonicate (5 min), filter and use the filtrate for spotting.

Chromatographic conditions :

Test plate : Hand-made TLC plate, coated with silica gel GF$_{254}$

Format : 10 × 10 cm   *Thickness :* 250 µm

Volume spotted : 10 µl   *Separation technique :* Ascending

Mobile phase :   1. Toluene–acetone (65 + 35, v/v)

2. Toluene–methanol–ammonia (75 + 25 + 0.25, v/v)

3. Toluene–chloroform–glacial acetic acid (100 + 50 + 10, v/v)

Chamber saturation : 30 min   *Migration distance :* 70 mm

Detection : UV (short) or iodine vapours or spray with 10% methanolic sulphuric acid and heat (105°C).

HRf :	1	2	3
Paracetamol	30	55	85
Oxyphenbutazone	60	35	55

Comments : —

Reference : —

PROTOCOLS OF A THIN LAYER CHROMATOGRAM

Chromatogram No. 73

Formulation : Paracetamol, Oxyphenbutazone
Classification : Analgesic and anti-inflammatory
Dosage form : Tablets
Standard solution : See Chromatogram No. 72.
Sample solution : See Chromatogram No. 72.
Chromatographic conditions :

Test plate : Hand-made TLC plate, coated with silica gel GF_{254} and impregnated with 5% silicone oil in petroleum ether (40-60).

Format : 10 × 10 cm   *Thickness :* 250 µm

Volume spotted : 10 µl   *Separation technique :* Ascending

Mobile phase : 0.5 M sodium chloride–methanol–glacial acetic acid (120 + 80 + 0.1, v/v)

Chamber saturation : —   *Migration distance :* 70 mm

Detection : UV (short) or iodine vapours

HRf : Paracetamol   75

         Oxyphenbutazone   50

Comments : See reversal of retention order as compared to normal-phase chromatography.
Reference : —

PROTOCOLS OF A THIN LAYER CHROMATOGRAM

Chromatogram No. 74

Formulation : **Oxyphenbutazone, Propyphenazone**

Classification : Analgesic and anti-inflammatory

Dosage form : Tablets

Standard solution : Prepare solution of each working standard in methanol for spotting.

Sample solution : Suspend powdered sample in methanol, sonicate, filter and use the filtrate for spotting.

Chromatographic conditions :

Test plate : Hand-made TLC plate, coated with silica gel GF$_{254}$ (activate at 105°C prior to use).

Format : 10 × 10 cm   *Thickness :* 250 μm

Volume spotted : 10 μl   *Separation technique :* Ascending

Mobile phase :   1. Toluene–acetone–glacial acetic acid (80 + 20 + 01, v/v)

2. Toluene–methanol–ammonia (75 + 25 + 0.25, v/v)

3. Butyl acetate–formic acid–chloroform (60 + 40 + 20, v/v)

4. Toluene–chloroform–glacial acetic acid (50 + 10 + 01, v/v)

Chamber saturation : 30 min   *Migration distance :* 70 mm

Detection : UV (short) or iodine vapours

HRf :

	1	2	3	4
Oxyphenbutazone	70	35	85	70
Propyphenazone	40	65	55	40

Comments : —

Reference : —

PROTOCOLS OF A THIN LAYER CHROMATOGRAM

Chromatogram No. 75

Formulation : Paracetamol, Chlorpheniramine maleate

Classification : Analgesic

Dosage form : Tablets

Standard solution : Prepare solution of each drug substance in methanol for spotting.

Sample solution : Extract powdered sample with methanol in ultrasonic water-bath, filter and use the filtrate for spotting.

Chromatographic conditions :

Test plate : Hand-made TLC plate, coated with silica gel GF_{254}

Format : 10 × 10 cm   *Thickness :* 250 μm

Volume spotted : 10 μl   *Separation technique :* Ascending

Mobile phase :   1. n-butanol–water–glacial acetic acid (80 + 20 + 20, v/v)

2. Chloroform–methanol–glacial acetic acid (100 + 20 + 20, v/v)

Chamber saturation : 30 min   *Migration distance :* 70 mm

Detection : UV (short) or iodine vapours

HRf :	1	2
Paracetamol	75	60
Chlorpheniramine maleate	30	15

Comments : —

Reference : —

PROTOCOLS OF A THIN LAYER CHROMATOGRAM

Chromatogram No. 76

Formulation : **Ibuprofen, Methocarbamol**

Classification : Analgesic and muscle relaxant

Dosage form : Tablets

Standard solution : Dissolve the working standard of each drug substance in methanol for spotting.

Sample solution : Suspend powdered sample in methanol, filter and use the filtrate.

Chromatographic conditions :

 Test plate : Pre-coated TLC plate, silica gel 60F$_{254}$

 Format : 10 × 10 cm   *Thickness :* 200 μm

 Volume spotted : 5 μl   *Separation technique :* Ascending

 Mobile phase : Toluene–ethyl acetate–glacial acetic acid (60 + 30 + 10, v/v)

 Chamber saturation : 30 min   *Migration distance :* 70 mm

 Detection : UV (short) or iodine vapours

 HRf : Ibuprofen   75

    Methocarbamol   30

Comments : —

Reference : —

Antibiotics

- Anti-tubercular drugs
- Penicillins
- Cephalosporins
- Antimalarials
- Anthelmintics
- Urinary antiseptics

PROTOCOLS OF A THIN LAYER CHROMATOGRAM

Chromatogram No. 77

Formulation : Isoniazid, Thiacetazone

Classification : Antibiotic (anti-tubercular)

Dosage form : Tablets/capsules

Standard solution : Prepare solution of each drug substance in methanol for application.

Sample solution : Extract the powdered sample with methanol by sonication. Centrifuge and use the supernatant for spotting.

Chromatographic conditions :

Test plate : Hand-made TLC plate, coated with silica gel GF$_{254}$ (activate at 105°C prior to use).

Format : 10 × 10 cm   *Thickness :* 250 µm

Volume spotted : 10 µl   *Separation technique :* Ascending

Mobile phase :   1. Toluene–methanol–ammonia (75 + 25 + 0.25, v/v)

2. Methanol–ammonia (200 + 03, v/v)

3. Butyl acetate–formic acid–chloroform (60 + 40 + 20, v/v)

4. Chloroform–methanol–glacial acetic acid (90 + 10 + 01, v/v)

Chamber saturation : 30 min   *Migration distance :* 70 mm

Detection : UV (short) or iodine vapours

HR*f* :	1	2	3	4
Isoniazid	30	40	15	30
Thiacetazone	65	65	60	45

Comments : —

Reference : —

PROTOCOLS OF A THIN LAYER CHROMATOGRAM

Chromatogram No. 78

Formulation : Isoniazid, Thiacetazone

Classification : Antibiotic (anti-tubercular)

Dosage form : Tablets/capsules

Standard solution : See Chromatogram No. 77.

Sample solution : See Chromatogram No. 77.

Chromatographic conditions :

Test plate : Hand-made TLC plate, coated with silica gel GF_{254} and impregnated with silicone oil in petroleum ether (40-60).

Format : 10 × 10 cm   *Thickness* : 250 μm

Volume spotted : 10 μl   *Separation technique* : Ascending

Mobile phase : 0.5 M sodium chloride–methanol–glacial acetic acid (120 + 80 + 0.1, v/v)

Chamber saturation : —   *Migration distance* : 70 mm

Detection : UV (short) or iodine vapours

HRf :   Isoniazid   60

      Thiacetazone   40

Comments : See reversal of retention order as compared to normal-phase chromatography.

Reference : —

PROTOCOLS OF A THIN LAYER CHROMATOGRAM

Formulation : Isoniazid, Ethambutol hydrochloride

Classification : Antibiotic (anti-tubercular)

Dosage form : Tablets

Standard solution : Dissolve each working standard in methanol for spotting.

Sample solution : Suspend powdered sample in methanol, sonicate for 10 min, filter and use the filtrate for spotting.

Chromatographic conditions :

Test plate : Hand-made TLC plate, coated with silica gel GF$_{254}$ (activate prior to use).

Format : 10 × 10 cm   *Thickness :* 250 μm

Volume spotted : 10 μl   *Separation technique :* Ascending

Mobile phase :   1. Methanol–ammonia (200 + 03, v/v)

2. Toluene–methanol–ammonia (75 + 25 + 0.25, v/v)

Chamber saturation : 30 min   *Migration distance :* 70 mm

Detection : UV (short)—only isoniazid; iodine vapours—both components

HRƒ :	1	2
Isoniazid	40 (70)*	30
Ethambutol hydrochloride	15 (30)*	15

* Without chamber saturation

Comments : After exposure to iodine vapours, ethambutol, a non-UV absorbing compound can also be detected under UV.

Reference : —

PROTOCOLS OF A THIN LAYER CHROMATOGRAM

Chromatogram No. 80

Formulation : **Isoniazid, Pyridoxine hydrochloride**

Classification : Antibiotic (anti-tubercular)

Dosage form : Tablets/capsules

Standard solution : Appropriate quantity of each working standard is dissolved in methanol for spotting.

Sample solution : The powdered sample is extracted with methanol by sonication. Filter and use the filtrate for spotting.

Chromatographic conditions :

Test plate : Hand-made TLC plate, coated with silica gel GF$_{254}$ (activate at 105°C prior to use).

Format : 10 × 10 cm   *Thickness* : 250 µm

Volume spotted : 10 µl   *Separation technique* : Ascending

Mobile phase :   1. Toluene–acetone–methanol–ammonia (25 + 70 + 05 + 01, v/v)

2. Toluene–methanol–ammonia (75 + 25 + 0.25, v/v)

3. Methanol–ammonia (200 + 03, v/v)

* 4. Acetone–carbon tetrachloride–6.5 M ammonia (21 + 07 + 02, v/v)

Chamber saturation : 30 min   *Migration distance* : 70 mm

Detection : UV (short) or iodine vapours

HRf :

	1	2	3
Isoniazid	50	30	40
Pyridoxine hydrochloride	30	40	60

Comments : —

Reference : * A.P. Argekar, S.S. Kunjir. J. Planar. Chromatography, 9, 390-394, 1996.

PROTOCOLS OF A THIN LAYER CHROMATOGRAM

Chromatogram No. 81

Formulation : Isoniazid, Pyrazinamide, Rifampicin

Classification : Antibiotic (anti-tubercular)

Dosage form : Tablets/capsules

Standard solution : Prepare solution of each working standard in methanol for spotting.

Sample solution : Suspend powdered sample in methanol, sonicate for 5 min, centrifuge and use the supernatant.

Chromatographic conditions :

Test plate : Hand-made TLC plate, coated with silica gel GF$_{254}$ (activate at 105°C prior to use).

Format : 10 × 20 cm   *Thickness :* 250 µm

Volume spotted : 10 µl   *Separation technique :* Ascending

Mobile phase : 1. Chloroform–methanol (90 + 10, v/v)
2. Toluene–methanol–ammonia (75 + 25 + 0.25, v/v)
3. Methanol–ammonia (200 + 03, v/v)

Chamber saturation : 30 min   *Migration distance :* 150 mm

Detection : UV (short) or iodine vapours

HRf :	1	2	3
Isoniazid	20	20	40
Pyrazinamide	50	30	55
Rifampicin	60	40	75

Comments : —

Reference : —

PROTOCOLS OF A THIN LAYER CHROMATOGRAM

Chromatogram No. 82

Formulation : Ampicillin, Cloxacillin sodium

Classification : Antibiotic

Dosage form : Capsules, suspension

Standard solution : Dissolve each drug substance in methanol for chromatography.

Sample solution : Suspend powdered sample in methanol, sonicate for 5 min, centrifuge and use the supernatant for spotting.

Chromatographic conditions :

Test plate : Hand-made TLC plate, coated with silica gel GF_{254} (activate at 105°C prior to use).

Format : 10 × 10 cm   *Thickness :* 250 μm

Volume spotted : 10 μl   *Separation technique :* Ascending

Mobile phase : Acetone–methanol–glacial acetic acid (50 + 45 + 05, v/v)

Chamber saturation : 30 min   *Migration distance :* 70 mm

Detection : Visible (spray with 0.2% ninhydrin solution in acetone, heat at 105°C for 10 min.)

HRf : Ampicillin   30
         Cloxacillin sodium   75

Comments : —

Reference : —

PROTOCOLS OF A THIN LAYER CHROMATOGRAM

Formulation : Ampicillin, Cloxacillin sodium

Classification : Antibiotic

Dosage form : Tablets, suspension

Standard solution : See Chromatogram No. 82.

Sample solution : See Chromatogram No. 82.

Chromatographic conditions :

Test plate : Reversed-phase TLC plate, silica gel KC-18F (Whatman)

Format : 10 × 10 cm   *Thickness :* 250 μm

Volume spotted : 5 μl   *Separation technique :* Ascending

Mobile phase : Methanol–0.1 M dipotassium hydrogen phosphate (55 + 45, v/v)

Chamber saturation : 30 min (paper lined) *Migration distance :* 70 mm

Detection : See Chromatogram No. 82.

HRf : Ampicillin   70

         Cloxacillin sodium   40

Comments : 1. See reversal of retention time in reversed-phase as compared to normal-phase.

2. On silica gel layer, there is possibility of degradation of β-lactam molecule, the use of RP-layer is recommended.

Reference : —

PROTOCOLS OF A THIN LAYER CHROMATOGRAM

Chromatogram No. 84

Formulation : Cephalexin, Probenecid

Classification : Antibiotic

Dosage form : Capsules

Standard solution : Prepare solution of each drug substance in methanol for spotting.

Sample solution : Appropriate quantity of powdered sample is extracted with methanol by sonication. Filter and use the filtrate for application.

Chromatographic conditions :

Test plate : Hand-made TLC plate, coated with silica gel GF$_{254}$

Format : 10 × 10 cm   *Thickness :* 250 μm

Volume spotted : 10 μl   *Separation technique :* Ascending

Mobile phase :   1. Chloroform–methanol–ammonia (70 + 25 + 0.7, v/v)

              * 2. Chloroform–methanol–ammonia (70 + 26 + 04, v/v)

Chamber saturation : 30 min   *Migration distance :* 70 mm

Detection : UV (short)

HRf :	1	2
Cephalexin	25	54
Probenecid	40	93

Comments : —

Reference : * U.P. Halkar and N.P. Bhandari. Indian Drugs, 35 (6), 382-383, 1998.

PROTOCOLS OF A THIN LAYER CHROMATOGRAM

Chromatogram No. 85

Formulation : Cephalexin, Probenecid

Classification : Antibiotic

Dosage form : Capsules

Standard solution : See Chromatogram No. 84.

Sample solution : See Chromatogram No. 84.

Chromatographic conditions :

Test plate : Hand-made TLC plate, coated with silica gel GF_{254}, impregnated with **5%** silicone oil in petroleum ether (40-60).

Format : 10×10 cm   *Thickness :* 250 µm

Volume spotted : 10 µl   *Separation technique :* Ascending

Mobile phase : 0.5 M sodium chloride–methanol–acetonitrile–glacial acetic acid (50 + 20 + 30 + 01, v/v)

Chamber saturation : —   *Migration distance :* 70 mm

Detection : UV (short)

HRf : Cephalexin   70

        Probenecid   40

Comments : Reversal of retention order in reversed-phase as compared to normal-phase.

Reference : —

PROTOCOLS OF A THIN LAYER CHROMATOGRAM

Chromatogram No. 86

Formulation : Gentamycin sulphate (C_1, C_{1a}, C_2, C_{2a})

Classification : Antibiotic

Dosage form : Eye/ear drops/injections

Standard solution : The antibiotic is dissolved in methanol–phosphate buffer (pH 8.0) 1 + 1.

Sample solution : Dilute appropriate volume of the sample with methanol–phosphate buffer (pH 8.0) 1 + 1 for spotting.

Chromatographic conditions :

Test plate : Reversed-phase pre-coated plate KC-8F or KC-18F (Whatman)

Format : 5 × 10 cm   *Thickness :* 200 μm

Volume spotted : 5 μl   *Separation technique :* Ascending

Mobile phase : 0.1 M lithium chloride in ammonia–methanol (100 + 20, v/v)

Chamber saturation : —   *Migration distance :* 70 mm

Detection : Post-chromatographic derivatization. After development, dry the plate in warm air. Spray with the reagent and heat at 110-120°C for 10-15 min, cool, spray with liquid paraffin solution. Observe fluorescent spots under UV (long) after 20-30 min.

Reagents : 1. Dissolve 35 mg of diphenyl boric anhydride and 25 mg of salicyl aldehyde in 100 ml of dichloromethane.

2. Prepare solution of liquid paraffin in n-hexane (1 : 6).

HRf :   Gentamycin C_1 30
       Gentamycin C_{1a} 55
       Gentamycin C_2 45
       Gentamycin C_{2a} 40

Comments : —

Reference : —

PROTOCOLS OF A THIN LAYER CHROMATOGRAM

Chromatogram No. 87

Formulation : Gentamycin sulphate (C_1, C_{1a}, C_2, C_{2a})

Classification : Antibiotic

Dosage form : Eye/ear drops/injections

Standard solution : See Chromatogram No. 86.

Sample solution : See Chromatogram No. 86.

Chromatographic conditions :

Test plate : Pre-coated TLC plate, silica gel $60F_{254}$ (pre-washed with methanol–chloroform 1 + 1 and dried at 105°C for 30 min)

Format : 10 × 10 cm   *Thickness :* 250 μm

Volume spotted : 5 μl   *Separation technique :* Ascending

Mobile phase : Chloroform–methanol–ammonia (1 + 1 + 1, v/v). Use lower organic **layer**.

Chamber saturation : Use twin-trough chamber, saturate with ammonia for 10 min   *Migration distance :* 70 mm

Detection : Visible, spray with 0.5% p-dimethyl amino cinnamaldehyde, heat at 100°C for 20 min and then expose the plate to ammonia vapours—red coloured spots against yellow background. Or spray with fluorescamine reagent and observe under UV (long). Or spray with 0.25% solution of ninhydrin and heat at 110°C for 5 min.

Reagent : Dissolve 0.5 g of PDAC in 50 ml of hydrochloric acid and dilute to 100 ml with methanol. Further dilute with methanol (1 + 1).

HRf :

Comments : —

Reference : —

PROTOCOLS OF A THIN LAYER CHROMATOGRAM

Chromatogram No. 88

Formulation : Neomycin sulphate (B, C) and Neamin (Neomycin A)

Classification : Antibiotic

Dosage form : Eye drops and ointment

Standard solution : Dissolve working standard of neomycin sulphate in 80% methanol.

Sample solution : Extract the ointment with 80% methanol, keep in freezer overnight and use the supernatant. Eye drops, if required, may be directly diluted with 80% methanol or used as such.

Chromatographic conditions :

Test plate : Pre-coated TLC plate, silica gel 60F$_{254}$

Format : 10 × 10 cm   *Thickness :* 200 μm

Volume spotted : 5 μl   *Separation technique :* Ascending

Mobile phase :   1. Methanol–ammonia–acetone–chloroform (70 + 40 + 40 + 10, v/v)

2. Methanol–acetone–5% acetic acid (120 + 150 + 130, v/v)

3. Methanol–acetone–ammonia (120 + 150 + 130, v/v)

4. Methanol–chloroform–ammonia (30 + 10 + 20, v/v)

Chamber saturation : —   *Migration distance :* 70 mm

Detection : UV (long) for fluorescent spots after post-chromatographic derivatization.

HRf :

Comments : Spray with fluorescamine solution and stabilize the spots by dipping the plate in solution of dichloromethane–triethanolamine–liquid paraffin (80 + 10 + 10). Fluorescent spots are visible after 30 min.

Reference :   1. Proc. International Symposium of Instrumental Chromatography, Interlaken, April 9-11, 69-73, 1997.

2. Adam E., et al. J. Pharm. Europa, 7 (2), 302-305, 1995.

PROTOCOLS OF A THIN LAYER CHROMATOGRAM

Chromatogram No. 89

Formulation : **Pyrimethamine/Sulphadoxine/Sulphamethoxypyridazine/Sulpha-methoxypyrazine**

Classification : Antibiotic (anti-malarial)

Dosage form : Tablets

Standard solution : Dissolve pyrimethamine in methanol and sulphonamide in methanol–ammonia (8 + 2) mixture.

Sample solution : Suspend the powdered sample in methanol–ammonia (8 + 2) mixture, sonicate for 5 min, centrifuge and use supernatant for spotting.

Chromatographic conditions :

Test plate : Hand-made TLC plate, coated with silica gel GF$_{254}$ (activate at 105°C prior to use).

Format : 20 × 20 cm   *Thickness* : 250 µm

Volume spotted : 10 µl   *Separation technique* : Ascending

Mobile phase : 1. Chloroform–methanol (120 + 05, v/v)

2. Toluene–methanol–ammonia (75 + 25 + 0.25, v/v)

3. Chloroform–methanol–DMF (100 + 10 + 05, v/v)

4. Toluene–ethyl acetate–acetone–ammonia (50 + 25 + 25 + 02, v/v)

Chamber saturation : 30 min   *Migration distance* : 150 mm

Detection : UV (short) or iodine vapours

HRf :

	1	2	3	4
Pyrimethamine	15	30	40	08
Sulphadoxine	35	50	60	50
Sulphamethoxypyridazine	40	—	55	30
Sulphamethoxypyrazine	50	—	—	—

Comments : —

Reference : —

PROTOCOLS OF A THIN LAYER CHROMATOGRAM

Chromatogram No. 90

Formulation : Dapsone, Clofazimine

Classification : Antibiotic (anti-leprotic)

Dosage form : Capsules

Standard solution : Initially dissolve each working standard in DMF. Further dilutions are made with methanol for spotting.

Sample solution : Suspend the powdered sample in DMF, vortex for 5 min, dilute with methanol, filter and use the filtrate for spotting.

Chromatographic conditions :

Test plate : Pre-coated TLC plate, coated with silica gel 60F$_{254}$

Format : 10 × 10 cm   *Thickness :* 250 μm

Volume spotted : 5 μl   *Separation technique :* Ascending

Mobile phase : Toluene–acetone (80 + 20, v/v)

Chamber saturation : 30 min   *Migration distance :* 70 mm

Detection : UV (short) or iodine vapours

HRf : Dapsone   20

       Clofazimine   35

Comments : —

Reference : —

PROTOCOLS OF A THIN LAYER CHROMATOGRAM

Formulation : Mebendazole, Pyrantel pamoate

Classification : Antibiotic (anthelmintic)

Dosage form : Tablets, suspension

Standard solution : Dissolve working standard of each substance in minimum quantity of DMF, and then dilute with methanol for spotting.

Sample solution : Initially extract the powdered sample with DMF and then dilute with methanol. Filter and use the filtrate for spotting.

Chromatographic conditions :

Test plate : Pre-coated TLC plate, silica gel 60F$_{254}$

Format : 10 × 10 cm   *Thickness :* 250 μm

Volume spotted : 10 μl   *Separation technique :* Ascending

Mobile phase :   Xylene–ethyl acetate–glacial acetic acid (50 + 50 + 02, v/v)

                    * Toluene–ethyl acetate–glacial acetic acid (50 + 50 + 02, v/v)

Chamber saturation : 30 min   *Migration distance :* 70 mm

Detection : UV (short) or iodine vapours

HRf :   1   2

     Mebendazole   55   65

     Pyrantel pamoate   15   20

Comments : —

Reference : * S.S. Zarapkar, et al. Indian Drugs, 35 (1), p. 49, 1998.

PROTOCOLS OF A THIN LAYER CHROMATOGRAM

Chromatogram No. 92

Formulation : Piperazine citrate, Diethylcarbamazine citrate

Classification : Antibiotic (anthelmintic)

Dosage form : Tablets

Standard solution : Dissolve each drug substance separately in 80% methanol.

Sample solution : Suspend the powdered sample in 80% methanol, shake for 5 min, filter and use the filtrate for spotting.

Chromatographic conditions :

Test plate : Hand-made TLC plate, coated with silica gel GF$_{254}$

Format : 10 × 20 cm   Thickness : 250 μm

Volume spotted : 10 μl   Separation technique : Ascending

Mobile phase : 1. Butyl acetate–formic acid–chloroform (60 + 40 + 20, v/v)
                         2. Methanol–ammonia (100 + 1.5, v/v)

Chamber saturation : —   Migration distance : 150 mm

Detection : Iodine vapours

HRf :	1	2
Piperazine citrate	10	05
Diethylcarbamazine citrate	40	50

Comments : —

Reference : —

PROTOCOLS OF A THIN LAYER CHROMATOGRAM

Chromatogram No. 93

Formulation : Diethylcarbamazine citrate, Chlorpheniramine maleate
Classification : Antibiotic (anthelmintic)
Dosage form : Tablets/syrup
Standard solution : See Chromatogram No. 92.
Sample solution : See Chromatogram No. 92.
Chromatographic conditions :

Test plate : Hand-made TLC plate, coated with silica gel GF$_{254}$ (activate at 105°C prior to use).

Format : 10 × 20 cm   *Thickness* : 250 μm

Volume spotted : 10 μl   *Separation technique* : Ascending

Mobile phase :   1. Butyl acetate–formic acid–chloroform (60 + 40 + 20, v/v)

          2. Methanol–ammonia (200 + 03, v/v)

Chamber saturation : 30 min   *Migration distance* : 150 mm

Detection : Iodine vapours

HRf :

	1	2
Diethylcarbamazine citrate	40	50
Chlorpheniramine maleate	25	30

Comments : —
Reference : —

PROTOCOLS OF A THIN LAYER CHROMATOGRAM

Chromatogram No. 94

Formulation : Phenolphthalein, Tetramisole hydrochloride

Classification : Antibiotic (anthelmintic)

Dosage form : Tablets

Standard solution : Prepare the solution of each drug substance in methanol for spotting.

Sample solution : Suspend the powdered sample in methanol, sonicate for 5 min, centrifuge and use the supernatant for spotting.

Chromatographic conditions :

Test plate : Hand-made TLC plate, coated with silica gel GF$_{254}$ (activate at 105°C prior to use).

Format : 10 × 20 cm   *Thickness :* 250 μm

Volume spotted : 10 μl   *Separation technique :* Ascending

Mobile phase : Butyl acetate–formic acid–chloroform (60 + 40 + 20, v/v)

Chamber saturation : 30 min   *Migration distance :* 150 mm

Detection :   1. Visible (spray with 1% alcoholic solution of sodium hydroxide)—phenol-phthalein

2. Iodine vapours (both substances)

HRf :   Phenolphthalein   75

Tetramisole hydrochloride   40

Comments : —

Reference : —

PROTOCOLS OF A THIN LAYER CHROMATOGRAM

Chromatogram No. 95

Formulation : Trimethoprim, Sulphamethoxazole/Sulphadiazine

Classification : Antibiotic (urinary anti-infective)

Dosage form : Tablets/capsules

Standard solution : The solution of all the drug substances was prepared in methanol for spotting.

Sample solution : Suspend the powdered sample in methanol and extract by slight warming. Filter and use the filtrate for spotting.

Chromatographic conditions :

Test plate : Hand-made TLC plate, coated with silica gel GF_{254} (activate at 105°C prior to use).

Format : 10 × 20 cm   *Thickness :* 250 μm

Volume spotted : 10 μl   *Separation technique :* Ascending

Mobile phase : 1. Chloroform–methanol–DMF (100 + 05 + 05, v/v)

　　　　　　　　 2. Toluene–ethyl acetate–acetone–ammonia (50 + 25 + 25 + 02, v/v)

　　　　　　　　 3. Chloroform–methanol (90 + 10, v/v)

Chamber saturation : 30 min   *Migration distance :* 150 mm

Detection : UV (short) or iodine vapours

HRf :	1	2	3
Trimethoprim	20	10	20
Sulphamethoxazole	45	60	50
Sulphadiazine	45	30	—

Comments : —

Reference : J.K. Lalla, et al. Indian Drugs, 34 (5), p. 275-282, 1997.

PROTOCOLS OF A THIN LAYER CHROMATOGRAM

Chromatogram No. 96

Formulation : Trimethoprim, Nitrofurantoin

Classification : Antibiotic (urinary anti-infective)

Dosage form : Tablets/capsules

Standard solution : See Chromatogram No. 95.

Sample solution : See Chromatogram No. 95.

Chromatographic conditions :

Test plate : Hand-made TLC plate, coated with silica gel GF$_{254}$ (activate at 105°C prior to use).

Format : 10 × 20 cm   *Thickness :* 250 μm

Volume spotted : 10 μl   *Separation technique :* Ascending

Mobile phase : Chloroform–methanol (95 + 05, v/v)

Chamber saturation : 30 min   *Migration distance :* 100 mm

Detection : UV (short), iodine vapours, nitrofurantoin visible as yellow spots

ḢRf : Trimethoprim   25

  Nitrofurantoin   35

Comments : —

Reference : —

PROTOCOLS OF A THIN LAYER CHROMATOGRAM

Formulation : Phenazopyridine hydrochloride, Nitrofurantoin

Classification : Antibiotic (urinary anti-infective)

Dosage form : Tablets

Standard solution : Dissolve working standard of each drug substance in methanol for spotting.

Sample solution : Suspend the powdered sample in methanol, sonicate for 10 min, centrifuge and use the supernatant for spotting.

Chromatographic conditions :

Test plate : Pre-coated TLC plate, silica gel 60F$_{254}$

Format : 10 × 10 cm   *Thickness :* 250 μm

Volume spotted : 5 μl   *Separation technique :* Ascending

Mobile phase : n-hexane–ethyl acetate–glacial acetic acid (50 + 50 + 01, v/v)

Chamber saturation : 30 min   *Migration distance :* 70 mm

Detection : UV (short), iodine vapours, nitrofurantoin visible as yellow spots

HRf : Nitrofurantoin   20

　　　 Phenazopyridine hydrochloride   45

Comments : —

Reference : —

PROTOCOLS OF A THIN LAYER CHROMATOGRAM

Chromatogram No. 98

Formulation : Trimethoprim, Nitrofurantoin, Phenazopyridine hydrochloride

Classification : Antibiotic (urinary anti-infective)

Dosage form : Tablets

Standard solution : See Chromatogram No. 97.

Sample solution : See Chromatogram No. 97.

Chromatographic conditions :

Test plate : Reversed-phase pre-coated TLC plate, silica gel 60RP-18F$_{254s}$

Format : 10 × 10 cm   *Thickness :* 250 μm

Volume spotted : 5 μl   *Separation technique :* Ascending

Mobile phase : 0.5 M sodium chloride–methanol–glacial acetic acid (120 + 80 + 01, v/v)

Chamber saturation : 30 min   *Migration distance :* 70 mm

Detection : UV (short); visible—phenazopyridine and nitrofurantoin

HRf :   Trimethoprim   40

       Nitrofurantoin   55

       Phenazopyridine hydrochloride   20

Comments : —

Reference : —

PROTOCOLS OF A THIN LAYER CHROMATOGRAM

Chromatogram No. 99

Formulation : Nalidixic acid, Metronidazole

Classification : Antibiotic (urinary anti-infective, anti-diarrhoeal)

Dosage form : Tablets, suspension

Standard solution : Prepare the solution of both the drug substances in methanol for spotting.

Sample solution : Extract the powdered sample with methanol by sonicating for 5-10 min. Filter and use the filtrate for spotting, dilute suspension with methanol, centrifuge and use the clear supernatant for spotting.

Chromatographic conditions :

Test plate : Pre-coated TLC plate, silica gel 60F$_{254}$

Format : 10 × 10 cm   *Thickness :* 250 µm

Volume spotted : 5 µl   *Separation technique :* Ascending

Mobile phase : Ethyl acetate–chloroform–methanol–ammonia (25 + 25 + 15 + 05, v/v)

Chamber saturation : 30 min   *Migration distance :* 70 mm

Detection : UV (short)

HRf :   Nalidixic acid   15

        Metronidazole   65

Comments : —

Reference : A.P. Argekar, et al. Indian Drugs, 33 (4), 167, 1996.

Central Nervous System

- **Sedatives and tranquillisers**
- **Anti-emetics and anti-nauseants**
- **Antimigraines**

PROTOCOLS OF A THIN LAYER CHROMATOGRAM

Chromatogram No. 100

Formulation : Imipramine hydrochloride, Diazepam

Classification : Sedative and tranquillizer

Dosage form : Tablets

Standard solution : Dissolve working standard of each substance in methanol for spotting.

Sample solution : Suspend appropriate quantity of the powdered sample in methanol, sonicate for 5 min, decant and use the clear solution for spotting.

Chromatographic conditions :

Test plate : Hand-made TLC plate, coated with silica gel GF$_{254}$ (activate at 105°C prior to use).

Format : 10 × 20 cm *Thickness :* 250 μm

Volume spotted : 10 μl *Separation technique :* Ascending

Mobile phase : 1. Toluene–methanol–ammonia (75 + 25 + 0.25, v/v)

2. Toluene–acetone–ammonia (70 + 30 + 01, v/v)

Chamber saturation : 30 min *Migration distance :* 100 mm

Detection : UV (short) or iodine vapours

HRf :	1	2
Imipramine hydrochloride	50	30
Diazepam	75	60

Comments : —

Reference : —

PROTOCOLS OF A THIN LAYER CHROMATOGRAM

Chromatogram No. 101

Formulation : Imipramine hydrochloride, Diazepam

Classification : Sedative and tranquillizer

Dosage form : Tablets

Standard solution : See Chromatogram No. 100.

Sample solution : See Chromatogram No. 100.

Chromatographic conditions :

Test plate : Reversed-phase pre-coated TLC plate, silica gel 60RP-18F$_{254s}$

Format : 10 × 10 cm   *Thickness :* 250 μm

Volume spotted : 5 μl   *Separation technique :* Ascending

Mobile phase : 0.5 M sodium chloride–methanol–acetonitrile–glacial acetic acid (50 + 20 + 30 + 01, v/v)

Chamber saturation : —   *Migration distance :* 70 mm

Detection : UV (short) or iodine vapours

HRf :   Imipramine hydrochloride   45

        Diazepam   30

Comments : See reversal of retention order as compared to normal-phase chromatography.

Reference : —

PROTOCOLS OF A THIN LAYER CHROMATOGRAM

Chromatogram No. 102

Formulation : **Trifluoperazine hydrochloride, Chlorpromazine, Trihexiphenidyl hydro-chloride**

Classification : Sedative and tranquillizer

Dosage form : Tablets/capsules

Standard solution : Prepare solution of each drug substance in methanol for spotting.

Sample solution : Extract the powdered sample in methanol in ultrasonic water-bath, decant and use the clear solution for spotting.

Chromatographic conditions :

Test plate : Hand-made TLC plate, coated with silica gel GF_{254}

Format : 10×20 cm   *Thickness :* 250 μm

Volume spotted : 10 μl   *Separation technique :* Ascending

Mobile phase : 1. Toluene–methanol–ammonia (75 + 25 + 0.25, v/v)

2. Toluene–acetone–methanol–ammonia (80 + 10 + 10 + 0.5, v/v)

Chamber saturation : 30 min   *Migration distance :* 150 mm

Detection : Iodine vapours—all components; UV (short)—trifluoperazine hydrochloride and chlorpromazine

HRf :

	1	2
Trifluoperazine hydrochloride	35	30
Chlorpromazine	55	60
Trihexiphenidyl hydrochloride	70	75

Comments : —

Reference : —

PROTOCOLS OF A THIN LAYER CHROMATOGRAM

Chromatogram No. 103

Formulation : Trifluoperazine hydrochloride, Promethazine hydrochloride, Isopropamide iodide

Classification : Sedative and tranquillizer

Dosage form : Tablets

Standard solution : See Chromatogram No. 102.

Sample solution : See Chromatogram No. 102.

Chromatographic conditions :

Test plate : Hand-made TLC plate, coated with silica gel GF$_{254}$ (activate at 105°C prior to use).

Format : 10 × 20 cm   *Thickness :* 250 µm

Volume spotted : 10 µl   *Separation technique :* Ascending

Mobile phase : Toluene–methanol–ammonia (75 + 25 + 0.25, v/v)

Chamber saturation : 30 min   *Migration distance :* 100 mm

Detection : Iodine vapours—all components; UV (short)—trifluoperazine hydrochloride and promethazine hydrochloride

HRf : Trifluoperazine hydrochloride   35

         Promethazine hydrochloride'   65

         Isopropamide iodide   20

Comments : —

Reference : —

PROTOCOLS OF A THIN LAYER CHROMATOGRAM

Chromatogram No. 104

Formulation : Chlordiazepoxide, Clidinium bromide

Classification : Sedative and tranquillizer

Dosage form : Tablets/capsules

Standard solution : Both the drug substances are separately dissolved in methanol for spotting.

Sample solution : Suspend powdered sample in methanol, vortex for 5 min, centrifuge and use the supernatant.

Chromatographic conditions :

Test plate : Hand-made TLC plate, coated with silica gel GF_{254} (activate at 105°C prior to use).

Format : 10 × 20 cm   *Thickness* : 250 μm

Volume spotted : 10 μl   *Separation technique* : Ascending

Mobile phase : Toluene–methanol–ammonia (75 + 25 + 0.25, v/v)

Chamber saturation : 30 min   *Migration distance* : 100 mm

Detection : Iodine vapours—all components; UV (short)—chlordiazepoxide

HRf : Chlordiazepoxide   70

         Clidinium bromide   10

Comments : —

Reference : —

PROTOCOLS OF A THIN LAYER CHROMATOGRAM

Chromatogram No. 105

Formulation : Chlordiazepoxide, Amitryptaline hydrochloride

Classification : Sedative and tranquillizer

Dosage form : Tablets/capsules

Standard solution : Prepare solution of both the substances in methanol for application.

Sample solution : Powdered sample is shaken with methanol, filtered and the filtrate used for spotting.

Chromatographic conditions :

Test plate : Pre-coated TLC plate, silica gel 60F$_{254}$

Format : 10 × 10 cm   *Thickness :* 250 μm

Volume spotted : 5 μl   *Separation technique :* Ascending

Mobile phase : 1. Ethyl acetate–methanol–diethylamine (95 + 05 + 0.5, v/v)
              2. Chloroform–methanol–ammonia (98 + 08 + 0.2, v/v)

Chamber saturation : 10 min   *Migration distance :* 70 mm

Detection : UV (short) or iodine vapours

HRf :	1	2
Chlordiazepoxide	60	40
Amitryptaline hydrochloride	30	55

Comments : —

Reference : —

PROTOCOLS OF A THIN LAYER CHROMATOGRAM

Chromatogram No. 106

Formulation : Chlordiazepoxide, Amitryptaline hydrochloride

Classification : Sedative and tranquillizer

Dosage form : Tablets/capsules

Standard solution : See Chromatogram No. 105.

Sample solution : See Chromatogram No. 105.

Chromatographic conditions :

Test plate : Reversed-phase pre-coated TLC plate, silica gel 60RP-18F$_{254s}$

Format : 10 × 10 cm   *Thickness* : 200 µm

Volume spotted : 5 µl   *Separation technique* : Ascending

Mobile phase : 0.5 M sodium chloride–methanol–acetonitrile–glacial acetic acid (50 + 20 + 30 + 01, v/v)

Chamber saturation : —   *Migration distance* : 70 mm

Detection : UV (short) or iodine vapours

HRf : Chlordiazepoxide   25

Amitryptaline hydrochloride   15

Comments : See reversal of retention order in reversed-phase chromatography as compared to normal phase chromatography.

Reference : —

PROTOCOLS OF A THIN LAYER CHROMATOGRAM

Chromatogram No. 107

Formulation : Haloperidol, Benzhexol

Classification : Sedative

Dosage form : Tablets

Standard solution : Prepare solution of each drug substance in chloroform for spotting.

Sample solution : Suspend the powdered sample in chloroform, sonicate, decant and use the clear solution for spotting.

Chromatographic conditions :

Test plate : Pre-coated TLC plate, silica gel GF$_{254}$

Format : 10 × 10 cm   *Thickness :* 250 μm

Volume spotted : 5 μl   *Separation technique :* Ascending

Mobile phase : Toluene–methanol–triethylamine (90 + 10 + 02, v/v)

Chamber saturation : 10 min   *Migration distance :* 70 mm

Detection : UV (short) or iodine vapours

HRf : Haloperidol   75

        Benzhexol   35

Comments : —

Reference : —

PROTOCOLS OF A THIN LAYER CHROMATOGRAM

Chromatogram No. 108

Formulation : Ergotamine tartrate, Caffeine citrate, Cyclizine hydrochloride
Classification : CNS (anti-emetic)
Dosage form : Tablets
Standard solution : Dissolve working standard of each analyte in methanol for spotting.
Sample solution : Powdered sample is suspended in methanol, vortexed for 5 min, supernatant used for spotting.
Chromatographic conditions :

Test plate : Hand-made TLC plate, coated with silica gel GF$_{254}$

Format : 10 × 20 cm   *Thickness :* 250 μm

Volume spotted : 10 μl   *Separation technique :* Ascending

Mobile phase : 1. Toluene–acetone–ammonia (40 + 60 + 02, v/v)

  2. Butyl acetate–formic acid–chloroform (60 + 40 + 20, v/v)

  3. Ethyl acetate–n-heptane–methanol–ammonia (60 + 30 + 7.5 + 02, v/v)

Chamber saturation : 25 min   *Migration distance :* 100 mm

Detection : Iodine vapours; UV (long)—ergotamine appears as fluorescent spot.

HRf :	1	2	3
Ergotamine tartrate	40	25	15
Caffeine citrate	55	50	45
Cyclizine hydrochloride	65	15	60

Comments : —
Reference : —

PROTOCOLS OF A THIN LAYER CHROMATOGRAM

Chromatogram No. 109

Formulation : Ergotamine tartrate, Caffeine citrate, Paracetamol, Prochlorperazine maleate

Classification : CNS (anti-emetic)

Dosage form : Tablets

Standard solution : See Chromatogram No. 108.

Sample solution : See Chromatogram No. 108.

Chromatographic conditions :

Test plate : Hand-made TLC plate, coated with silica gel GF$_{254}$ (activate at 105°C prior to use).

Format : 10 × 20 cm   *Thickness :* 250 μm

Volume spotted : 10 μl   *Separation technique :* Ascending

Mobile phase : Butyl acetate–formic acid–chloroform (60 + 40 + 20, v/v)

Chamber saturation : 30 min   *Migration distance :* 150 mm

Detection : Iodine vapours

HRf :		
	Ergotamine tartrate	25
	Caffeine citrate	50
	Paracetamol	65
	Prochlorperazine maleate	10

Comments : —

Reference : —

PROTOCOLS OF A THIN LAYER CHROMATOGRAM

Chromatogram No. 110

Formulation : Meclozine hydrochloride, Caffeine citrate, Pyridoxine hydrochloride
Classification : CNS (anti-emetic)
Dosage form : Tablets
Standard solution : See Chromatogram No. 108.
Sample solution : See Chromatogram No. 108.
Chromatographic conditions :

Test plate : Hand-made TLC plate, coated with silica gel GF_{254} (activate at 105°C prior to use).

Format : 10 × 20 cm   *Thickness :* 250 μm

Volume spotted : 10 μl   *Separation technique :* Ascending

Mobile phase :   1. Toluene–acetone–glacial acetic acid (60 + 13 + 01, v/v)
                         2. Toluene–methanol–acetone–ammonia (150 + 50 + 50 + 01, v/v)
                         3. Toluene–methanol–ammonia (75 + 25 + 0.25, v/v)

Chamber saturation : 30 min   *Migration distance :* 100 mm

Detection : UV (short) or iodine vapours

HRf :

	1	2	3
Meclozine hydrochloride	45	75	70
Caffeine citrate	20	40	50
Pyridoxine hydrochloride			30

Comments : —
Reference : —

PROTOCOLS OF A THIN LAYER CHROMATOGRAM

Chromatogram No. 111

Formulation : Meclozine hydrochloride, Hydroxyzine hydrochloride, Nicotinic acid
Classification : CNS (anti-emetic)
Dosage form : Tablets
Standard solution : See Chromatogram No. 108.
Sample solution : See Chromatogram No. 108.
Chromatographic conditions :

Test plate : Hand-made TLC plate, coated with silica gel GF$_{254}$ (activate at 105°C prior to use).

Format : 10 × 20 cm   *Thickness :* 250 μm

Volume spotted : 10 μl   *Separation technique :* Ascending

Mobile phase : Toluene–methanol–ammonia (75 + 25 + 0.25, v/v)

Chamber saturation : 20 min   *Migration distance :* 100 mm

Detection : UV (short) or iodine vapours

HRf :   Meclozine hydrochloride   70
        Hydroxyzine hydrochloride   55
        Nicotinic acid   05

Comments : —
Reference : —

PROTOCOLS OF A THIN LAYER CHROMATOGRAM

Chromatogram No. 112

Formulation : Pyridoxine hydrochloride, Prochlorperazine maleate
Classification : CNS (anti-emetic)
Dosage form : Tablets
Standard solution : See Chromatogram No. 108.
Sample solution : See Chromatogram No. 108.
Chromatographic conditions :

Test plate : Pre-coated TLC plate, silica gel 60F$_{254}$

Format : 10 × 20 cm   *Thickness* : 250 μm

Volume spotted : 10 μl   *Separation technique* : Ascending

Mobile phase : Toluene–methanol–ammonia (75 + 25 + 0.25, v/v)

Chamber saturation : 15 min   *Migration distance* : 100 mm

Detection : UV (short) or iodine vapours

HRf : Pyridoxine hydrochloride   30

Prochlorperazine maleate   60

Comments : —
Reference : —

Alimentary System

- **Anti-diarrhoeals**
- **Anti-spasmodics**

PROTOCOLS OF A THIN LAYER CHROMATOGRAM

Chromatogram No. 113

Formulation : Metronidazole, Diloxanide furoate, Furazolidone

Classification : Alimentary drugs (anti-diarrhoeal)

Dosage form : Tablets, suspension

Standard solution : Prepare solution of each working standard in chloroform for spotting.

Sample solution : Suspend the sample in chloroform. Sonicate for 5-10 min, decant and use the clear solution for spotting.

Chromatographic conditions :

Test plate : Hand-made TLC plate, coated with silica gel GF$_{254}$ (activate at 105°C prior to use).

Format : 10 × 20 cm   *Thickness :* 250 μm

Volume spotted : 10 μl   *Separation technique :* Ascending

Mobile phase : 1. Toluene–acetone–ammonia (80 + 20 + 05, v/v)
 2. Toluene–methanol–ammonia (75 + 25 + 0.25, v/v)
 3. Ethyl acetate–chloroform (100 + 100, v/v)
 4. Dichloromethane–methanol (96 + 04, v/v)
 5. Chloroform–acetone–methanol (100 + 16 + 04, v/v)
 6. Toluene–ethyl acetate–methanol (60 + 35 + 05, v/v)

Chamber saturation : 25 min   *Migration distance :* 100 mm

Detection : UV (short) or iodine vapours

HRf :

	1	2	3	4	5	6
Metronidazole	10	20	20	35	35	22
Diloxanide furoate	60	75	75	80	—	84
Furazolidone	—	50	50	—	65	35

Comments : —

Reference : —

PROTOCOLS OF A THIN LAYER CHROMATOGRAM

Chromatogram No. 114

Formulation : Tinidazole/Metronidazole, Diloxanide furoate, Furazolidone

Classification : Alimentary drugs (anti-diarrhoeal)

Dosage form : Tablets, suspension

Standard solution : See Chromatogram No. 113.

Sample solution : See Chromatogram No. 113.

Chromatographic conditions :

Test plate : Hand-made TLC plate, coated with silica gel GF$_{254}$ (activate at 105°C prior to use).

Format : 10 × 20 cm   *Thickness :* 250 μm

Volume spotted : 10 μl   *Separation technique :* Ascending

Mobile phase :   1. Toluene–methanol–ammonia (75 + 25 + 0.25, v/v)

  2. Toluene–acetone–ammonia (80 + 20 + 05, v/v)

  3. Chloroform–methanol–ammonia (90 + 10 + 01, v/v)

  4. Chloroform–acetone–methanol–ammonia (100 + 15 + 05 + 01, v/v)

Chamber saturation : 30 min   *Migration distance :* 150 mm

Detection : UV (short), iodine vapours

HRf :

	1	2	3	4
Tinidazole	85	15	75	65
Diloxanide furoate	75	60	—	—
Furazolidone	50	60	60	55
Metronidazole	20	10	—	—

PROTOCOLS OF A THIN LAYER CHROMATOGRAM

Chromatogram No. 115

Formulation : Tinidazole, Norfloxacin

Classification : Alimentary drugs (anti-diarrhoeal)

Dosage form : Tablets, suspension

Standard solution : Dissolve both the substances in methanol–dichloromethane (1 + 1).

Sample solution : Suspend the sample in methanol–dichloromethane (1 + 1), shake for 5-10 min, filter and use the filtrate for spotting.

Chromatographic conditions :

Test plate : Pre-coated TLC plate, silica gel GF_{254} (pre-wash with ammoniacal methanol)

Format : 10 × 10 cm   *Thickness :* 250 μm

Volume spotted : 5 μl   *Separation technique :* Ascending

Mobile phase :   1. Chloroform–methanol–toluene–diethylamine–water (40 + 40 + 20 + 14 + 08, v/v)

2. n-butanol–ethyl acetate–ammonia (40 + 10 + 0.2, v/v)

Chamber saturation : 15 min   *Migration distance :* 70 mm

Detection : UV (short)

HRf :

	1	2
Tinidazole	75	80
Norfloxacin	45	40

Comments : —

Reference : —

PROTOCOLS OF A THIN LAYER CHROMATOGRAM

Chromatogram No. 116

Formulation : Sennoside A, B, C, D

Classification : Alimentary drugs

Dosage form : Tablets

Standard solution : Dissolve the sennoside standard in methanol for spotting.

Sample solution : For extraction of sample, use the soxhlet extraction procedure using methanol.

Chromatographic conditions :

Test plate : Pre-coated TLC plate, SIL N-HR-UV$_{254}$

Format : 10 × 10 cm   *Thickness :* 200 μm

Volume spotted : 5 μl   *Separation technique :* Ascending

Mobile phase : Iso-propanol–ethyl acetate–water (36 + 36 + 28, v/v)

Chamber saturation : —   *Migration distance :* 50 mm

Detection : Visible and UV (long)

HRf :   Sennoside A   20

          Sennoside B   35

          Sennoside C   55

          Sennoside D   45

Comments : —

Reference : TLC Application Notes (M & N), p. A-18.

PROTOCOLS OF A THIN LAYER CHROMATOGRAM

Chromatogram No. 117

Formulation : Ethylmorphine, Dicyclomine hydrochloride
Classification : Alimentary drugs (anti-spasmodic)
Dosage form : Tablets
Standard solution : Dissolve both the substances in methanol for spotting.
Sample solution : Suspend the powdered sample in methanol, sonicate for 5 min, centrifuge and use the supernatant for spotting.
Chromatographic conditions :

Test plate : TLC pre-coated plate, silica gel 60F$_{254}$

Format : 10 × 10 cm   *Thickness :* 250 μm

Volume spotted : 5 μl   *Separation technique :* Ascending

Mobile phase : Toluene–acetone–methanol–ammonia (7 + 2 + 1 + 0.05, v/v)

Chamber saturation : 30 min   *Migration distance :* 70 mm

Detection : Visible, iodine vapours

HRf :   Ethylmorphine   25
          Dicyclomine hydrochloride   60

Comments : After developing, the plate is sprayed with diluted reagent and air dried, blue spots are observed.

Spray reagent : Dissolve 6.06 g of potassium thiocyanate, 50 g of cobalt (II) chloride, 3.4 g of sodium acetate in 20 ml of water, add 2.5 ml of 1 M HCl and dilute to 25 ml with water. Dilute 10 ml of this reagent to 125 ml with methanol and use as spray reagent.

Reference : —

PROTOCOLS OF A THIN LAYER CHROMATOGRAM

Chromatogram No. 118

Formulation : Analgin, Baralgan amide, Baralgan ketone

Classification : Alimentary drugs (anti-spasmodic)

Dosage form : Tablets

Standard solution : Dissolve working standard of each analyte in methanol for application.

Sample solution : Extract the powdered sample with chloroform–methanol (1 + 4), filter, evaporate the filtrate and take up the residue in methanol for spotting.

Chromatographic conditions :

Test plate : Pre-coated TLC plate, silica gel 60F$_{254}$

Format : 10 × 10 cm	*Thickness :* 250 µm
Volume spotted : 5 µl	*Separation technique :* Ascending

Mobile phase : Toluene–methanol–ammonia (75 + 25 + 0.25, v/v)

Chamber saturation : 30 min	*Migration distance :* 70 mm

Detection : UV—analgin and baralgan ketone; Dragendorff's reagent—baralgan amide and ketone

HRf :   Analgin   20
   Baralgan amide   20
   Baralgan ketone 50

Comments : First observe under UV for analgin and ketone, then spray with the reagent; amide and ketone appear as orange spot against yellow background.

Reference : —

PROTOCOLS OF A THIN LAYER CHROMATOGRAM

Chromatogram No. 119

Formulation : **Atropine methonitrate, Papaverine hydrochloride, Paracetamol, Chlorpromazine hydrochloride**

Classification : Alimentary drugs (anti-spasmodic)

Dosage form : Tablets

Standard solution : Dissolve all the drug substances in chloroform–methanol (1 + 3) for spotting.

Sample solution : Shake the powdered sample with chloroform–methanol (1 + 3), use the supernatant for spotting.

Chromatographic conditions :

Test plate : Hand-made TLC plate, coated with silica gel GF_{254}

Format : 10 × 20 cm   Thickness : 250 μm

Volume spotted : 10 μl   Separation technique : Ascending

Mobile phase : Butyl acetate–formic acid–chloroform (60 + 40 + 2, v/v)

Chamber saturation : 30 min   Migration distance : 100 mm

Detection : UV (short) or iodine vapours

HRf :   Atropine methonitrate   15

Papaverine hydrochloride   35

Paracetamol   55

Chlorpromazine hydrochloride   45

Comments : —

Reference : —

PROTOCOLS OF A THIN LAYER CHROMATOGRAM

Chromatogram No. 120

Formulation : Atropine sulphate, Scopolamine (Hyoscine)

Classification : Alimentary drugs (anti-spasmodic)

Dosage form : Tablets

Standard solution : Prepare the solution of working standard of each drug in methanol for application.

Sample solution : Extract the powdered sample with methanol by shaking, filter and use the filtrate for spotting.

Chromatographic conditions :

Test plate : Reversed-phase pre-coated TLC plate, silica gel 60RP-18F$_{254s}$

Format : 10 × 10 cm   *Thickness :* 250 μm

Volume spotted : 5 μl   *Separation technique :* Ascending

Mobile phase : 0.5 M sodium chloride–acetone (60 + 40, v/v)

Chamber saturation : —   *Migration distance :* 70 mm

Detection : UV (254), iodine vapours or spray with Dragendorff's reagent

HRf : Atropine sulphate   70

        Scopolamine (Hyoscine)   80

Comments : —

Reference : Application Manual on HPLC/TLC/HPTLC, p. 138, E. Merck.

Respiratory System

- Expectorants
- Antitussives
- Mucolytics
- Bronchodilators (anti-asthma)
- Anti-allergic drugs

PROTOCOLS OF A THIN LAYER CHROMATOGRAM

Chromatogram No. 121

Formulation : **Ephedrine hydrochloride, Pseudoephedrine hydrochloride, Triprolidine hydrochloride**

Classification : Respiratory system (anti-asthma)

Dosage form : Tablets/capsules

Standard solution : Prepare solution of working standard of each drug substance in methanol for spotting.

Sample solution : Suspend powdered sample in methanol, shake, filter and use the filtrate for spotting.

Chromatographic conditions :

Test plate : Hand-made TLC plate, coated with silica gel GF$_{254}$ (activate at 105°C prior to use).

Format : 10 × 20 cm   *Thickness :* 250 μm

Volume spotted : 10 μl   *Separation technique :* Ascending

Mobile phase : 1. Toluene–methanol–ammonia (75 + 25 + 0.25, v/v)

2. Chloroform–methanol–ammonia (100 + 05 + 0.5, v/v)

3. Butyl acetate–formic acid–chloroform (60 + 40 + 20, v/v)

Chamber saturation : 30 min   *Migration distance :* 100 mm

Detection : Iodine vapours or spray with 0.1% ninhydrin solution and heat at 105°C for localization of spots.

HRf :

	1	2	3
Ephedrine hydrochloride	15	10	45
Pseudoephedrine hydrochloride	20	10	45
Triprolidine hydrochloride	40	20	10

Comments : —

Reference : —

PROTOCOLS OF A THIN LAYER CHROMATOGRAM

Chromatogram No. 122

Formulation : Ephedrine hydrochloride, Pseudoephedrine hydrochloride, Triprolidine hydrochloride

Classification : Respiratory system (anti-asthma)

Dosage form : Tablets

Standard solution : See Chromatogram No. 121.

Sample solution : See Chromatogram No. 121.

Chromatographic conditions :

Test plate : Reversed-phase pre-coated TLC plate, silica gel 60RP-18F$_{254s}$

Format : 10 × 10 cm   *Thickness :* 250 μm

Volume spotted : 5 μl   *Separation technique :* Ascending

Mobile phase : 0.5 M sodium chloride–methanol–acetonitrile–glacial acetic acid (50 + 20 + 30 + 01, v/v)

Chamber saturation : —   *Migration distance :* 70 mm

Detection : Iodine vapours or spray with 0.1% ninhydrin solution

HRf :   Ephedrine hydrochloride   55

           Pseudoephedrine hydrochloride   60

           Triprolidine hydrochloride   20

Comments : —

Reference : —

PROTOCOLS OF A THIN LAYER CHROMATOGRAM

Chromatogram No. 123

Formulation : **Betamethasone, Chlorpheniramine maleate**

Classification : Respiratory system (anti-allergic)

Dosage form : Tablets

Standard solution : Prepare solution of both the analytes in methanol for spotting.

Sample solution : Extract the powdered sample with methanol, filter and use the filtrate for spotting.

Chromatographic conditions :

Test plate : Hand-made TLC plate, coated with silica gel GF_{254} (activate at 105°C **prior** to use).

Format : 10×20 cm   *Thickness :* 250 μm

Volume spotted : 10 μl   *Separation technique :* Ascending

Mobile phase : Toluene–methanol–ammonia (75 + 25 + 0.25, v/v)

Chamber saturation : 20 min   *Migration distance :* 100 mm

Detection : UV (short) or iodine vapours

HRf :   Betamethasone   20

        Chlorpheniramine maleate   35

Comments : —

Reference : —

PROTOCOLS OF A THIN LAYER CHROMATOGRAM

Chromatogram No. 124

Formulation : Dexamethasone, Cyproheptadine hydrochloride

Classification : Respiratory system (anti-allergic)

Dosage form : Tablets/capsules

Standard solution : Solution of both the drug substances is prepared in methanol for spotting.

Sample solution : Extract the powdered sample with methanol in ultrasonic water-bath, filter and use the filtrate for spotting.

Chromatographic conditions :

Test plate : Pre-coated TLC plate, silica gel 60F$_{254}$

Format : 10 × 10 cm   Thickness : 250 μm

Volume spotted : 5 μl   Separation technique : Ascending

Mobile phase : 1. Toluene–methanol–ammonia (75 + 25 + 0.25, v/v)

                2. Butyl acetate–formic acid–chloroform (60 + 40 + 20, v/v)

Chamber saturation : 15 min   Migration distance : 70 mm

Detection : UV (short) or iodine vapours

HRƒ :	1	2
Dexamethasone	30	45
Cyproheptadine hydrochloride	50	60

Comments : —

Reference : —

PROTOCOLS OF A THIN LAYER CHROMATOGRAM

Chromatogram No. 125

Formulation : Chlorpheniramine maleate, Trithioparamethoxyphenylpropene

Classification : Respiratory system (anti-allergic)

Dosage form : Tablets

Standard solution : Dissolve working standard of both the drug substances in methanol for spotting.

Sample solution : The powdered sample is extracted with methanol by sonication. Filter and use the filtrate for spotting.

Chromatographic conditions :

Test plate : Pre-coated TLC plate, silica gel 60F$_{254}$

Format : 10 × 10 cm   *Thickness :* 250 μm

Volume spotted : 5 μl   *Separation technique :* Ascending

Mobile phase : Cyclohexane–toluene–diethylamine (75 + 15 + 03, v/v)

Chamber saturation : —   *Migration distance :* 70 mm

Detection : Visible—trithioparamethoxyphenylpropene; UV (short)—both the components

HRf : Chlorpheniramine maleate   20

Trithioparamethoxyphenylpropene   35

Comments : —

Reference : —

PROTOCOLS OF A THIN LAYER CHROMATOGRAM

Chromatogram No. 126

Formulation : Terfenadine, Terfenadinone

Classification : Respiratory system (anti-allergic)

Dosage form : Tablets

Standard solution : See Chromatogram No. 125.

Sample solution : See Chromatogram No. 125.

Chromatographic conditions :

Test plate : Pre-coated TLC plate, silica gel $60F_{254}$

Format : 10 × 10 cm   *Thickness :* 250 µm

Volume spotted : 5 µl   *Separation technique :* Ascending

Mobile phase : Chloroform–ethyl acetate–methanol–ammonia (70 + 80 + 10 + 10, v/v)

Chamber saturation : 30 min   *Migration distance :* 70 mm

Detection : UV (short) or iodine vapours

HRf :   Terfenadine   45

       Terfenadinone   70

Comments : —

Reference : —

PROTOCOLS OF A THIN LAYER CHROMATOGRAM

Chromatogram No. 127

Formulation : Cetirizine hydrochloride, Chlorpheniramine maleate
Classification : Respiratory system (anti-allergic)
Dosage form : Tablets
Standard solution : See Chromatogram No. 125.
Sample solution : See Chromatogram No. 125.
Chromatographic conditions :

Test plate : Pre-coated TLC plate, silica gel 60F$_{254}$

Format : 10 × 10 cm   *Thickness :* 250 µm

Volume spotted : 5 µl   *Separation technique :* Ascending

Mobile phase : Toluene–ethyl acetate–methanol–ammonia (35 + 50 + 15 + 3.0, v/v)

Chamber saturation : 10 min   *Migration distance :* 70 mm

Detection : UV (short) or iodine vapours

HRf :   Cetirizine hydrochloride   10
          Chlorpheniramine maleate   45

Comments : —
Reference : —

PROTOCOLS OF A THIN LAYER CHROMATOGRAM

Chromatogram No. 128

Formulation : Pseudoephedrine hydrochloride, Azatadine maleate, Paracetamol

Classification : Respiratory system (anti-allergic)

Dosage form : Tablets

Standard solution : Dissolve all the drug substances in methanol for spotting.

Sample solution : Suspend the powdered sample in methanol, sonicate for 10 min, filter and use the filtrate for spotting.

Chromatographic conditions :

Test plate : Pre-coated TLC plate, silica gel 60F$_{254}$

Format : 10 × 10 cm   *Thickness :* 250 μm

Volume spotted : 5 μl   *Separation technique :* Ascending

Mobile phase : Dichloromethane–acetone–methanol–triethylamine (70 + 40 + 50 + 02, v/v)

Chamber saturation : 10 min   *Migration distance :* 70 mm

Detection : UV (short) or iodine vapours

HRf :   Pseudoephedrine hydrochloride   25

          Azatadine maleate   35

          Paracetamol   75

Comments : —

Reference : Jyoti Chawla, Renu Sodhi and R.T. Sane. Indian Drugs, 33 (5), 208-212, 1996.

PROTOCOLS OF A THIN LAYER CHROMATOGRAM

Chromatogram No. 129

Formulation : Theophylline, Salbutamol sulphate

Classification : Respiratory system (anti-asthma)

Dosage form : Syrup

Standard solution : Dissolve both the drug substances in methanol containing small amount of ammonia for spotting.

Sample solution : Dilute the sample with methanol containing small amount of ammonia, cool in refrigerator and use the supernatant for spotting.

Chromatographic conditions :

Test plate : Hand-made TLC plate, coated with silica gel GF_{254} (activate at 105°C prior to use).

Format : 10 × 10 cm   *Thickness :* 250 μm

Volume spotted : 10 μl   *Separation technique :* Ascending

Mobile phase : 1. Toluene–methanol–ammonia (75 + 25 + 0.25, v/v)
                    2. Methanol–ammonia (100 + 03, v/v)

Chamber saturation : 20 min   *Migration distance :* 70 mm

Detection : UV (short) or iodine vapours

HRf :

	1	2
Theophylline	10	30
Salbutamol sulphate	40	70

Comments : —

Reference : —

PROTOCOLS OF A THIN LAYER CHROMATOGRAM

Chromatogram No. 130

Formulation : Theophylline, Etofylline

Classification : Respiratory system (anti-asthma)

Dosage form : Tablets/syrup

Standard solution : See Chromatogram No. 129.

Sample solution : See Chromatogram No. 129.

Chromatographic conditions :

  Test plate : Pre-coated TLC plate, silica gel 60F$_{254}$

  Format : 10 × 10 cm   *Thickness :* 250 µm

  Volume spotted : 5 µl   *Separation technique :* Ascending

  Mobile phase : 1. Chloroform–acetone–glacial acetic acid (80 + 20 + 02, v/v)

    2. Chloroform–methanol (90 + 10, v/v)

  Chamber saturation : 10 min   *Migration distance :* 70 mm

  Detection : UV (short) or iodine vapours

  HRf :

	1	2
Theophylline	45	60
Etofylline	28	45

Comments : —

Reference : —

PROTOCOLS OF A THIN LAYER CHROMATOGRAM

Chromatogram No. 131

Formulation : Theophylline, Ephedrine hydrochloride, Hydroxyzine hydrochloride

Classification : Respiratory system (anti-asthma)

Dosage form : Tablets, syrup

Standard solution : Prepare solution of ephedrine hydrochloride and hydroxyzine hydrochloride in methanol and theophylline in ammonia, mix together to get analyte solution for spotting.

Sample solution : Shake sample with ammonia–water (1 + 2), vortex and dilute with methanol. Filter and use the filtrate for spotting.

Chromatographic conditions :

Test plate : Hand-made TLC plate, coated with silica gel GF$_{254}$

Format : 10 × 20 cm   *Thickness :* 250 µm

Volume spotted : 10 µl   *Separation technique :* Ascending

Mobile phase :   1. Toluene–methanol–ammonia (75 + 25 + 0.25, v/v)

               2. Ethyl acetate–methanol–ammonia (100 + 15 + 0.5, v/v)

Chamber saturation : 30 min   *Migration distance :* 100 mm

Detection : UV (short) or iodine vapours

HRf :

	1	2
Theophylline	40	40
Ephedrine hydrochloride	15	10
Hydroxyzine hydrochloride	70	70

Comments : —

Reference : —

PROTOCOLS OF A THIN LAYER CHROMATOGRAM

Chromatogram No. 132

Formulation : Theophylline, Hydroxyzine hydrochloride, Terbutaline sulphate

Classification : Respiratory system (anti-asthma)

Dosage form : Tablets, syrup

Standard solution : See Chromatogram No. 131.

Sample solution : See Chromatogram No. 131.

Chromatographic conditions :

Test plate : Pre-coated TLC plate, silica gel $60F_{254}$

Format : 10×10 cm   *Thickness :* 250 μm

Volume spotted : 5 μl   *Separation technique :* Ascending

Mobile phase : 1. Toluene–methanol–ammonia (75 + 25 + 0.25, v/v)

  2. Chloroform–acetone–methanol–ammonia (40 + 10 + 05 + 01, v/v)

Chamber saturation : 10 min   *Migration distance :* 70 mm

Detection : UV (short) or iodine vapours

HRf :

	1	2
Theophylline	40	35
Hydroxyzine hydrochloride	10	10
Terbutaline sulphate	70	60

Comments : —

Reference : —

PROTOCOLS OF A THIN LAYER CHROMATOGRAM

Chromatogram No. 133

Formulation : Theophylline, Ephedrine hydrochloride, Phenobarbitone, Chlorpheniramine maleate

Classification : Respiratory system (anti-asthma)

Dosage form : Tablets, syrup

Standard solution : Dissolve working standard of each drug substance in methanol for spotting.

Sample solution : See Chromatogram No. 131.

Chromatographic conditions :

Test plate : Hand-made TLC plate, coated with silica gel GF$_{254}$ (activate prior to use).

Format : 10 × 20 cm   *Thickness :* 250 μm

Volume spotted : 10 μl   *Separation technique :* Ascending

Mobile phase : Toluene–methanol–ammonia (75 + 25 + 0.25, v/v)

Chamber saturation : 30 min   *Migration distance :* 100 mm

Detection : UV (short)—all components except ephedrine hydrochloride; iodine vapours. Spray with 0.1% ninhydrin solution followed by heating at 100°C to localize ephedrine hydrochloride.

HRf :   Theophylline   40
         Ephedrine hydrochloride   15
         Phenobarbitone   60
         Chlorpheniramine maleate   30

Comments : —

Reference : —

PROTOCOLS OF A THIN LAYER CHROMATOGRAM

Chromatogram No. 134

Formulation : Theophyllin ethonate of piperazine, Ephedrine hydrochloride, Phenobarbitone, Chlorpheniramine maleate, Guaiphenesin

Classification : Respiratory system (anti-asthma)

Dosage form : Syrup

Standard solution : See Chromatogram No. 133.

Sample solution : Basify the sample with ammonia, extract with chloroform, evaporate the chloroform layer and take up the residue in methanol for spotting.

Chromatographic conditions :

Test plate : Hand-made TLC plate, coated with silica gel GF$_{254}$ (activate prior to use)

Format : 20 × 20 cm   *Thickness :* 250 μm

Volume spotted : 10 μl   *Separation technique :* Ascending

Mobile phase : Toluene–methanol–ammonia (75 + 25 + 0.25, v/v)

Chamber saturation : 30 min   *Migration distance :* 100 mm

Detection : Iodine vapours

HRf :

Theophyllin ethonate of piperazine	05
Ephedrine hydrochloride	15
Phenobarbitone	60
Chlorpheniramine maleate	30
Guaiphenesin	40

Comments : —

Reference : —

PROTOCOLS OF A THIN LAYER CHROMATOGRAM

Chromatogram No. 135

Formulation : Salbutamol sulphate, Guaiphenesin, Chlorpheniramine maleate

Classification : Respiratory system (anti-asthma)

Dosage form : Syrup

Standard solution : Dissolve both the substances in methanol for spotting.

Sample solution : To appropriate quantity of syrup, add 2-3 drops of ammonia, 2-3 ml of methanol and 5 ml of acetone, keep in refrigerator for 2-3 hrs. Decant, evaporate and take up the residue in methanol.

Chromatographic conditions :

Test plate : Hand-made TLC plate, coated with silica gel GF$_{254}$

Format : 10×20 cm   *Thickness :* 250 μm

Volume spotted : 10 μl   *Separation technique :* Ascending

Mobile phase :   1. Toluene–methanol–ammonia $(75 + 25 + 0.25,$ v/v)

                      2. Butyl acetate–formic acid–chloroform $(60 + 40 + 20,$ v/v)

                      3. Chloroform–acetone–methanol–ammonia $(40 + 10 + 05 + 01,$ v/v)

Chamber saturation : 30 min   *Migration distance :* 100 mm

Detection : UV (short) or iodine vapours

HRf :	1	2	3
Salbutamol sulphate	10	20	15
Guaiphenesin	40	40	50
Chlorpheniramine maleate	30	30	30

Comments : —

Reference : —

PROTOCOLS OF A THIN LAYER CHROMATOGRAM

Chromatogram No. 136

Formulation : Salbutamol sulphate, Bromhexine hydrochloride, Chlorpheniramine maleate

Classification : Respiratory system (expectorant)

Dosage form : Syrup

Standard solution : See Chromatogram No. 135.

Sample solution : See Chromatogram No. 135.

Chromatographic conditions :

Test plate : Hand-made TLC plate, coated with silica gel GF$_{254}$ (activate prior to use).

Format : 10 × 20 cm   *Thickness :* 250 µm

Volume spotted : 10 µl   *Separation technique :* Ascending

Mobile phase :   1. Toluene–methanol–ammonia (75 + 25 + 0.25, v/v)

2. Butyl acetate–formic acid–chloroform (60 + 40 + 20, v/v)

3. Methanol–ammonia (200 + 03, v/v)

Chamber saturation : 30 min   *Migration distance :* 100 mm

Detection : Iodine vapours, UV (short)

HRf :

	1	2	3
Salbutamol sulphate	10	20	55
Bromhexine hydrochloride	65	60	75
Chlorpheniramine maleate	30	30	40

Comments : —

Reference : —

PROTOCOLS OF A THIN LAYER CHROMATOGRAM

Chromatogram No. 137

Formulation : Guaiphenesin sulphate, Phenylpropanolamine hydrochloride, Diphenyl-pyraline, Paracetamol

Classification : Respiratory system (expectorant)

Dosage form : Tablets, syrup

Standard solution : Prepare appropriate concentration of all the drug substances in methanol for spotting.

Sample solution : Concentrate the syrup over water-bath, add methanol, keep in refrigerator for 2-3 hrs., decant and use the clear solution.

Chromatographic conditions :

Test plate : Hand-made TLC plate, coated with silica gel GF_{254} (activate prior to use).

Format : 10 × 20 cm   *Thickness :* 250 μm

Volume spotted : 10 μl   *Separation technique :* Ascending

Mobile phase :   1. n-hexane–diethyl ether–methanol (30 + 30 + 40, v/v)

　　　　　　　 2. Toluene–methanol–ammonia (75 + 25 + 0.25, v/v)

　　　　　　　 3. Toluene–acetone–ammonia (50 + 50 + 02, v/v)

Chamber saturation : 30 min   *Migration distance :* 100 mm

Detection : Iodine vapours

HRf :	1	2	3
Guaiphenesin sulphate	60	45	30
Phenylpropanolamine hydrochloride	40	35	55
Diphenylpyraline	50	75	75
Paracetamol	70	55	20

Comments : —

Reference : —

PROTOCOLS OF A THIN LAYER CHROMATOGRAM

Chromatogram No. 138

Formulation : Guaiphenesin sulphate, Dexchlorpheniramine maleate, Pseudoephedrine hydrochloride

Classification : Respiratory system (expectorant)

Dosage form : Syrup

Standard solution : See Chromatogram No. 137.

Sample solution : See Chromatogram No. 137.

Chromatographic conditions :

Test plate : Hand-made TLC plate, coated with silica gel GF_{254} (activate prior to use).

Format : 10 × 20 cm   *Thickness :* 250 µm

Volume spotted : 10 µl   *Separation technique :* Ascending

Mobile phase :   1. Toluene–methanol–ammonia (75 + 25 + 0.25, v/v)

                * 2. Ethyl acetate–methanol–ammonia (170 + 20 + 10, v/v)

Chamber saturation : 30 min   *Migration distance :* 100 mm

Detection : Iodine vapours

HRf :   Guaiphenesin sulphate   45

           Dexchlorpheniramine maleate   35

           Pseudoephedrine hydrochloride   20

Comments : —

Reference : * M.P. Lippstone, et al. J. Plan. Chromatogr., 9, 456-458, 1996.

PROTOCOLS OF A THIN LAYER CHROMATOGRAM

Formulation : **Guaiphenesin sulphate, Chlorpheniramine maleate, Dextromethorphan hydrobromide**

Classification : Respiratory system (expectorant)

Dosage form : Syrup

Standard solution : See Chromatogram No. 137.

Sample solution : See Chromatogram No. 137.

Chromatographic conditions :

   Test plate : Hand-made TLC plate, coated with silica gel GF$_{254}$ (activate prior to use).

   Format : 10 × 20 cm   *Thickness* : 250 μm

   Volume spotted : 10 μl   *Separation technique* : Ascending

   Mobile phase : Toluene–methanol–ammonia (75 + 25 + 0.25, v/v)

   Chamber saturation : 30 min   *Migration distance* : 100 mm

   Detection : Iodine vapours

   HRf : Guaiphenesin sulphate   45

            Chlorpheniramine maleate   30

            Dextromethorphan hydrobromide   35

Comments : —

Reference : —

PROTOCOLS OF A THIN LAYER CHROMATOGRAM

Chromatogram No. 140

Formulation : Bromhexine hydrochloride, Ephedrine hydrochloride, Pseudoephedrine hydrochloride, Dextromethorphan hydrobromide

Classification : Respiratory system (expectorant)

Dosage form : Syrup

Standard solution : See Chromatogram No. 137.

Sample solution : See Chromatogram No. 137.

Chromatographic conditions :

Test plate : Hand-made TLC plate, coated with silica gel GF_{254} (activate prior to use).

Format : 10 × 20 cm   *Thickness :* 250 μm

Volume spotted : 10 μl   *Separation technique :* Ascending

Mobile phase : 1. Toluene–methanol–ammonia (75 + 25 + 0.25, v/v)

                        2. Ethylene dichloride–methanol–formic acid (75 + 25 + 05, v/v)

Chamber saturation : 30 min   *Migration distance :* 100 mm

Detection : Iodine vapours

HRf :	1	2
Bromhexine hydrochloride	65	30
Ephedrine hydrochloride	15	40
Pseudoephedrine hydrochloride	20	45
Dextromethorphan hydrobromide	35	—

Comments : —

Reference : —

PROTOCOLS OF A THIN LAYER CHROMATOGRAM

Chromatogram No. 141

Formulation : Dextromethorphan hydrobromide, Doxylamine succinate
Classification : Respiratory system (expectorant)
Dosage form : Syrup
Standard solution : —
Sample solution : —
Chromatographic conditions :

Test plate : Pre-coated TLC plate, silica gel $60F_{254}$

Format : 10×10 cm

Thickness : 250 μm

Volume spotted : 5 μl

Separation technique : Ascending

Mobile phase : Methanol–ammonia (140 + 10, v/v)

Chamber saturation : —

Migration distance : 70 mm

Detection : UV (short)

HRf : —

Comments : —

Reference : G. Indryanto. J. Planar Chromatography, 9, 282, 1996.

PROTOCOLS OF A THIN LAYER CHROMATOGRAM

Chromatogram No. 142

Formulation : **Ephedrine hydrochloride, Pseudoephedrine hydrochloride, Chlorpheniramine maleate, Noscapine, Aspirin, Caffeine citrate**

Classification : Respiratory system (expectorant)

Dosage form : Syrup

Standard solution : See Chromatogram No. 140.

Sample solution : See Chromatogram No. 140.

Chromatographic conditions :

Test plate : Hand-made TLC plate, coated with silica gel GF$_{254}$ (activate prior to use).

Format : 20 × 20 cm   *Thickness :* 250 µm

Volume spotted : 10 µl   *Separation technique :* Ascending

Mobile phase : Toluene–methanol–ammonia (75 + 25 + 0.25, v/v)

Chamber saturation : 30 min   *Migration distance :* 100 mm

Detection : UV (short). Spray with ninhydrin reagent followed by heating (105°C) to locate ephedrine and pseudoephedrine.

HRf :

Ephedrine hydrochloride	15
Pseudoephedrine hydrochloride	20
Chlorpheniramine maleate	30
Noscapine	80
Aspirin	10
Caffeine citrate	65

Comments : —

Reference : —

PROTOCOLS OF A THIN LAYER CHROMATOGRAM

Chromatogram No. 143

Formulation : Noscapine, Phenylpropanolamine hydrochloride, Paracetamol

Classification : Respiratory system (expectorant)

Dosage form : Syrup

Standard solution : Prepare solution of all the working standards in chloroform–methanol (8 + 2) for spotting.

Sample solution : Concentrate the syrup over water-bath and extract with chloroform–methanol (8 + 2) and use the supernatant for spotting.

Chromatographic conditions :

Test plate : Hand-made TLC plate, coated with silica gel 60F$_{254}$ (activate prior to use).

Format : 10 × 20 cm   *Thickness :* 250 μm

Volume spotted : 10 μl   *Separation technique :* Ascending

Mobile phase : Toluene–methanol–ammonia (75 + 25 + 0.25, v/v)

Chamber saturation : 30 min   *Migration distance :* 100 mm

Detection : Iodine vapours

HRf : Noscapine   80
         Phenylpropanolamine hydrochloride   35
         Paracetamol   55

Comments : —

Reference : —

PROTOCOLS OF A THIN LAYER CHROMATOGRAM

Chromatogram No. 144

Formulation : **Ephedrine hydrochloride, Codeine phosphate, Chlorpheniramine maleate, Promethazine hydrochloride**

Classification : Respiratory system (expectorant)

Dosage form : Syrup

Standard solution : See Chromatogram No. 143.

Sample solution : See Chromatogram No. 143.

Chromatographic conditions :

Test plate : Hand-made TLC plate, coated with silica gel GF$_{254}$ (activate prior to use).

Format : 20 × 20 cm   *Thickness :* 250 μm

Volume spotted : 10 μl   *Separation technique :* Ascending

Mobile phase :   1. Toluene–methanol–ammonia (75 + 25 + 0.25, v/v)

2. Butyl acetate–formic acid–chloroform (60 + 40 + 20, v/v)

Chamber saturation : 30 min   *Migration distance :* 100 mm

Detection : Iodine vapours

HRf :	1	2
Ephedrine hydrochloride	15	45
Codeine phosphate	40	20
Chlorpheniramine maleate	30	30
Promethazine hydrochloride	70	70

Comments : —

Reference : —

PROTOCOLS OF A THIN LAYER CHROMATOGRAM

Chromatogram No. 145

Formulation : Codeine phosphate, Chlorpheniramine maleate, Guaiphenesin sulphate
Classification : Respiratory system (expectorant)
Dosage form : Syrup
Standard solution : See Chromatogram No. 143.
Sample solution : See Chromatogram No. 143.
Chromatographic conditions :

Test plate : Hand-made TLC plate, coated with silica gel GF$_{254}$ (activate prior to use).

Format : 10 × 20 cm   *Thickness :* 250 μm

Volume spotted : 10 μl   *Separation technique :* Ascending

Mobile phase : Butyl acetate–formic acid–chloroform (60 + 40 + 20, v/v)

Chamber saturation : 30 min   *Migration distance :* 100 mm

Detection : Iodine vapours

HRf :   Codeine phosphate   20

            Chlorpheniramine maleate   30

            Guaiphenesin sulphate   40

Comments : —
Reference : —

PROTOCOLS OF A THIN LAYER CHROMATOGRAM

Chromatogram No. 146

Formulation : Diphenylpyraline hydrochloride, Phenylephrine hydrochloride, Para-cetamol

Classification : Respiratory system (expectorant)

Dosage form : Syrup

Standard solution : See Chromatogram No. 143.

Sample solution : See Chromatogram No. 143.

Chromatographic conditions :

Test plate : Hand-made TLC plate, coated with silica gel GF_{254} (activate prior to use).

Format : 10 × 20 cm   *Thickness :* 250 μm

Volume spotted : 10 μl   *Separation technique :* Ascending

Mobile phase : n-butyl alcohol–ammonia (80 + 20, v/v)

Chamber saturation : 30 min   *Migration distance :* 100 mm

Detection : Iodine vapours

HRf :   Diphenylpyraline hydrochloride   75

         Phenylephrine hydrochloride   40

         Paracetamol   55

Comments : —

Reference : —

PROTOCOLS OF A THIN LAYER CHROMATOGRAM

Chromatogram No. 147

Formulation : Pseudoephedrine hydrochloride, Dextromethorphan hydrobromide, Carbinoxamine maleate, Paracetamol

Classification : Respiratory system (expectorant)

Dosage form : Syrup

Standard solution : See Chromatogram No. 127.

Sample solution : See Chromatogram No. 127.

Chromatographic conditions :

Test plate : Hand-made TLC plate, coated with silica gel GF$_{254}$

Format : 20 × 20 cm   *Thickness :* 250 μm

Volume spotted : 10 μl   *Separation technique :* Ascending

Mobile phase : Ethyl acetate–acetone–ammonia (50 + 50 + 20, v/v)

Chamber saturation : 30 min   *Migration distance :* 100 mm

Detection : Iodine vapours

HRf : Pseudoephedrine hydrochloride   75

Dextromethorphan hydrobromide   25

Carbinoxamine maleate   35

Paracetamol   65

Comments : —

Reference : —

PROTOCOLS OF A THIN LAYER CHROMATOGRAM

Chromatogram No. 148

Formulation : **Phenylpropanolamine hydrochloride, Pheniramine maleate, Mepyramine maleate, Caffeine citrate**

Classification : Respiratory system (expectorant)

Dosage form : Syrup

Standard solution : See Chromatogram No. 143.

Sample solution : See Chromatogram No. 143.

Chromatographic conditions :

Test plate : Pre-coated TLC plate, silica gel 60F$_{254}$

Format : 10 × 10 cm   *Thickness :* 250 μm

Volume spotted : 5 μl   *Separation technique :* Ascending

Mobile phase : Toluene–methanol–ammonia (75 + 25 + 0.25, v/v)

Chamber saturation : 20 min   *Migration distance :* 100 mm

Detection : UV (short) or iodine vapours

HRf :   Phenylpropanolamine hydrochloride   35

      Pheniramine maleate   45

      Mepyramine maleate   55

      Caffeine citrate   70

Comments : —

Reference : —

Topical Preparations

- Antifungal drugs
- Anti-infective drugs
- Keratolytics and cleansers
- Rubefacients

PROTOCOLS OF A THIN LAYER CHROMATOGRAM

Chromatogram No. 149

Formulation : Salicylic acid, Lactic acid

Classification : Topical preparation

Dosage form : Lotion

Standard solution : Take up both the chemicals in methanol for spotting.

Sample solution : Dilute the lotion suitably with methanol for application.

Chromatographic conditions :

Test plate : Hand-made pre-coated TLC plate, SIL G-25 (activate at 105°C prior to use).

Format : 10 × 10 cm   *Thickness :* 250 µm

Volume spotted : 5 µl   *Separation technique :* Ascending

Mobile phase :   1. n-phenyl formate–chloroform–formic acid (70 + 15 + 15, v/v) or (20 + 70 + 10, v/v)

           2. Diisopropyl ether–formic acid–water (90 + 07 + 03, v/v)

Chamber saturation : 10 min   *Migration distance :* 70 mm

Detection : Spray with 1% methanolic solution of bromocresol green—yellow spots against light blue background

HRf :   Salicylic acid   70

        Lactic acid   35

Comments : —

Reference : TLC Application Notes (M & N), p. A-8, 1996.

PROTOCOLS OF A THIN LAYER CHROMATOGRAM

Chromatogram No. 150

Formulation : Salicylic acid, Benzoic acid, Resorcinol

Classification : Topical preparation

Dosage form : Lotion, ointment

Standard solution : Dissolve working standards of all the substances in chloroform or methanol for spotting.

Sample solution : Extract the sample (ointment) with methanol with slight warming, cool and use the supernatant.

Chromatographic conditions :

Test plate : Hand-made TLC plate, coated with silica gel GF_{254} (activate prior to use).

Format : 10×20 cm *Thickness :* 250 μm

Volume spotted : 10 μl *Separation technique :* Ascending

Mobile phase : 1. Chloroform–methanol (85 + 15, v/v)
2. n-hexane–acetic acid (96 + 04, v/v)
3. Ethyl acetate–acetone (90 + 20, v/v)

Chamber saturation : 30 min *Migration distance :* 100 mm

Detection : UV (short) or iodine vapours or spray with ferric chloride solution

HRf :	1	2	3
Salicylic acid	10	45	40
Benzoic acid	55	60	60
Resorcinol	70	05	—

Comments : —

Reference : —

PROTOCOLS OF A THIN LAYER CHROMATOGRAM

Chromatogram No. 151

Formulation : Salicylic acid, Dithranol

Classification : Topical preparation

Dosage form : Lotion, ointment, cream

Standard solution : See Chromatogram No. 150.

Sample solution : See Chromatogram No. 150.

Chromatographic conditions :

Test plate : Pre-coated TLC plate, silica gel $60F_{254}$

Format : 10×10 cm   *Thickness :* 250 µm

Volume spotted : 5 µl   *Separation technique :* Ascending

Mobile phase : n-hexane–ethyl acetate–glacial acetic acid (95 + 05 + 01, v/v)

Chamber saturation : 15 min   *Migration distance :* 70 mm

Detection : UV (short) or iodine vapours or spray with ferric chloride solution

HRf : Salicylic acid   15

      Dithranol   50

Comments : —

Reference : —

PROTOCOLS OF A THIN LAYER CHROMATOGRAM

Chromatogram No. 152

Formulation : Benzoic acid, Miconazole nitrate

Classification : Topical preparation

Dosage form : Cream, lotion

Standard solution : Dissolve both the substances in methanol for spotting.

Sample solution : Extract the sample with methanol with slight warming. (Freeze overnight in case of cream.) Cool and use the supernatant.

Chromatographic conditions :

Test plate : Pre-coated TLC plate, silica gel 60F$_{254}$

Format : 10 × 10 cm   *Thickness :* 250 μm

Volume spotted : 5 μl   *Separation technique :* Ascending

Mobile phase : n-hexane–chloroform–methanol–diethylamine (42 + 21 + 13 + 05, v/v)

Chamber saturation : —   *Migration distance :* 70 mm

Detection : UV (short) or iodine vapours

HRf : Benzoic acid   40

       Miconazole nitrate   65

Comments : —

Reference : —

PROTOCOLS OF A THIN LAYER CHROMATOGRAM

Formulation : Miconazole nitrate, Clotrimazole, Tinidazole

Classification : Topical preparation

Dosage form : Cream, vaginal tablets

Standard solution : See Chromatogram No. 152.

Sample solution : See Chromatogram No. 152.

Chromatographic conditions :

Test plate : Pre-coated TLC plate, silica gel 60F$_{254}$

Format : 10 × 10 cm   Thickness : 250 μm

Volume spotted : 5 μl   Separation technique : Ascending

Mobile phase : Toluene–acetone–ammonia (70 + 30 + 01, v/v)

Chamber saturation : 30 min   Migration distance : 70 mm

Detection : UV (short) or iodine vapours

HRf :   Miconazole nitrate   40

Clotrimazole   55

Tinidazole   25

Comments : —

Reference : —

PROTOCOLS OF A THIN LAYER CHROMATOGRAM

Chromatogram No. 154

Formulation : Miconazole nitrate, Clotrimazole, Betamethasone dipropionate

Classification : Topical preparation

Dosage form : Cream, lotion

Standard solution : Prepare solution of each substance in chloroform for spotting.

Sample solution : Suspend the sample in chloroform, shake for 10 min, use supernatant for application.

Chromatographic conditions :

Test plate : Pre-coated TLC plate, silica gel 60F$_{254}$

Format : 10 × 10 cm   *Thickness :* 250 μm

Volume spotted : 5 μl   *Separation technique :* Ascending

Mobile phase : Toluene–acetone–ammonia (70 + 30 + 01, v/v)

Chamber saturation : 20 min   *Migration distance :* 70 mm

Detection : UV (short) or iodine vapours

HRf :   Miconazole nitrate   40

      Clotrimazole   55

      Betamethasone dipropionate   65

Comments : —

Reference : —

PROTOCOLS OF A THIN LAYER CHROMATOGRAM

Chromatogram No. 155

Formulation : Miconazole nitrate, Hydrocortisone acetate

Classification : Topical preparation

Dosage form : Cream, lotion

Standard solution : See Chromatogram No. 154.

Sample solution : See Chromatogram No. 154.

Chromatographic conditions :

Test plate : Pre-coated TLC plate, silica gel $60F_{254}$

Format : 10×10 cm   *Thickness :* 250 µm

Volume spotted : 5 µl   *Separation technique :* Ascending

Mobile phase : Toluene–acetone–ammonia (70 + 30 + 01, v/v)

Chamber saturation : 10 min   *Migration distance :* 70 mm

Detection   UV (short) or iodine vapours

HRf :   Miconazole nitrate   40

        Hydrocortisone acetate   35

Comments : —

Reference : —

PROTOCOLS OF A THIN LAYER CHROMATOGRAM

Chromatogram No. 156

Formulation : Tolnaftate, Betamethasone valerate, Iodochlorhydroxyquinoline, Gentamycin

Classification : Topical preparation

Dosage form : Cream, lotion

Standard solution : Prepare solution of each substance in DMF–methanol (1 + 1), mix and use for application.

Sample solution : Extract the sample with DMF–methanol (1 + 1), keep in refrigerator (2 hrs.), use supernatant for spotting.

Chromatographic conditions :

Test plate : Pre-coated TLC plate, silica gel SIL G-25 [pre-wash with methanol–ammonia (50 + 1) prior to use].

Format : 10 × 10 cm   *Thickness :* 250 µm

Volume spotted : 5 µl   *Separation technique :* Ascending

Mobile phase : 1. Dichloromethane–diethyl ether–methanol–water (77 + 15 + 08 + 1.2, v/v)

2. Chloroform–acetone (60 + 20, v/v)

Chamber saturation : 20 min   *Migration distance :* 70 mm

Detection : UV (short). Spray with ninhydrin reagent for detection of gentamycin.

HRf :		
	Tolnaftate	65
	Betamethasone valerate	30
	Iodochlorhydroxyquinoline	50
	Gentamycin	05

Comments : —

Reference : Ethyl acetate–n-butanol–ammonia (110 + 50 + 40, v/v) may be used as mobile phase for preparations containing nipagin and nipasol (J. Planar. Chromatogr., 10, 204-207, 1997).

PROTOCOLS OF A THIN LAYER CHROMATOGRAM

Chromatogram No. 157

Formulation : Hydrocortisone, Cinchocaine

Classification : Topical preparation

Dosage form : Ointment, cream

Standard solution : Dissolve both the substances in methanol for spotting.

Sample solution : To appropriate quantity of the sample, add methanol, heat on a hot plate, cool and use the supernatant for application.

Chromatographic conditions :

Test plate : Hand-made/pre-coated HPTLC plate, silica gel 60F$_{254}$

Format : 10 × 10 cm   *Thickness :* 100 μm

Volume spotted : 4 μl   *Separation technique :* Ascending

Mobile phase : Toluene–acetone–acetic acid–ethanol (40 + 30 + 05 + 02, v/v)

Chamber saturation : 15 min   *Migration distance :* 65 mm

Detection : UV (short)

HRf : Hydrocortisone   25

          Cinchocaine   65

Comments : —

Reference : Application Notes, CBS-79, Sept. 97.

PROTOCOLS OF A THIN LAYER CHROMATOGRAM

Chromatogram No. 158

Formulation : Triamcinolone acetonide, Fluocinolone acetonide

Classification : Topical preparation

Dosage form : Ointment, lotion, cream

Standard solution : Prepare solution of each substance in methanol–dichloromethane (1 + 9).

Sample solution : The sample is shaken with methanol–dichloromethane (1 + 9), store in refrigerator and use supernatant for spotting.

Chromatographic conditions :

Test plate : Pre-coated TLC plate, silica gel SIL G-25 (pre-wash with methanol)

Format : 20 × 20 cm   *Thickness :* 250 µm

Volume spotted : 5 µl   *Separation technique :* Ascending

Mobile phase : Glacial acetic acid–carbon tetrachloride–heptane (40 + 30 + 30, v/v)

Chamber saturation : 30 min   *Migration distance :* 100 mm

Detection : UV (short) or spray with 5% methanolic sulphuric acid, heat at 105°C for 10 min and examine under long UV (365 nm).

HRf :		
	Triamcinolone	10
	Triamcinolone acetonide	35
	Fluocinolone acetonide	30
	Betamethasone	20
	Betamethasone acetate	45
	Betamethasone valerate	50
	Betamethasone dipropionate	75

Comments : —

Reference : J. Planar Chromatography, 6, 269-273, 1993.

PROTOCOLS OF A THIN LAYER CHROMATOGRAM

Chromatogram No. 159

Formulation : Capsaicin

Classification : Topical preparation

Dosage form : Cream, ointment

Standard solution : Suspend the oleo-resin in methanol or ethyl acetate for spotting.

Sample solution : Extract the sample with ethyl acetate by sonicating for 5 min, use the supernatant.

Chromatographic conditions :

Test plate : Pre-coated HPTLC plate, nano-SIL UV$_{254}$ (M & N)

Format : 5 × 5 cm   *Thickness :* 100 μm

Volume spotted : 1 μl   *Separation technique :* Ascending

Mobile phase :   1. Toluene–acetone–chloroform (40 + 35 + 25, v/v)

                   2. Toluene–methanol (90 + 10, v/v)

Chamber saturation : 30 min   *Migration distance :* 30 mm

Detection : UV (short) or spray with Gibb's reagent

HRf :   1   2

         Capsaicin   65   30

Comments : —

Reference : TLC Application Notes (M & N), p. A-12.

PROTOCOLS OF A THIN LAYER CHROMATOGRAM

Chromatogram No. 160

Formulation : Benzocaine, Chloramphenicol, 2-amino-1(4-nitrophenyl) propane-1,3-diol (ANDP)

Classification : Topical preparation

Dosage form : Ear drops, solution

Standard solution : Standard solution of all the substances was prepared in methanol for spotting.

Sample solution : Dilute the sample with methanol for spotting.

Chromatographic conditions :

Test plate : Pre-coated TLC plate, silica gel SIL-G25

Format : 10 × 10 cm　　　　　　　　*Thickness :* 250 μm

Volume spotted : 5 μl　　　　　　　*Separation technique :* Ascending

Mobile phase :　1. Toluene–acetone (75 + 25, v/v)

　　　　　　　　　2. n-butanol (water saturated)–glacial acetic acid (90 + 10, v/v)

Chamber saturation : 20 min　　　　*Migration distance :* 70 mm

Detection : UV (short)

HRf :

	1	2
Benzocaine	40	30
Chloramphenicol	20	80
ANDP	—	60

Comments : —

Reference : —

PROTOCOLS OF A THIN LAYER CHROMATOGRAM

Chromatogram No. 161

Formulation : **Chloramphenicol, Dexamethasone/Prednisolone/Betamethasone sodium phosphate**

Classification : Topical preparation

Dosage form : Eye/ear drops

Standard solution : Dissolve the substances in water–triethylamine (1 + 1) for spotting.

Sample solution : Dilute the sample with water–triethylamine.

Chromatographic conditions :

Test plate : Hand-made TLC plate, coated with mixed slurry of silianized silica gel H & HF$_{254}$ (1 + 1). Shake 5 g of each silica gel with 10 ml of methanol and 15 ml water for 2 min and coat the plate (activate at 105°C for 60 min prior to use).

Format : 10 × 20 cm   *Thickness :* 250 µm

Volume spotted : 10 µl   *Separation technique :* Ascending

Mobile phase : 0.05 M triethylamine (pH 4.2)–methanol (60 + 40, v/v)

Chamber saturation : 60 min   *Migration distance :* 100 mm

Detection : UV (short)

HRf :   Chloramphenicol   55
         Dexamethasone sodium phosphate   30
         Prednisolone sodium phosphate   30
         Betamethasone sodium phosphate   45

Comments : —

Reference : —

PROTOCOLS OF A THIN LAYER CHROMATOGRAM

Chromatogram No. 162

Formulation : Benzocaine, Hexylresorcinol, Antipyrine

Classification : Topical preparation

Dosage form : Ear drops

Standard solution : Prepare the solution of each working standard in methanol for spotting.

Sample solution : Directly dilute the spots with methanol for application.

Chromatographic conditions :

Test plate : Pre-coated TLC plate, silica gel SIL-G25

Format : 10 × 10 cm   *Thickness :* 250 μm

Volume spotted : 5 μl   *Separation technique :* Ascending

Mobile phase : Toluene–acetone (70 + 30, v/v)

Chamber saturation : 10 min   *Migration distance :* 70 mm

Detection : UV (short) or iodine vapours

HRf :   Benzocaine   40

      Hexylresorcinol   30

      Antipyrine   15

Comments : —

Reference : —

Miscellaneous Preparations

PROTOCOLS OF A THIN LAYER CHROMATOGRAM

Chromatogram No. 163

Formulation : Glycerin, Ethylene glycol, Propylene glycol, Diethylene glycol
Classification : Miscellaneous
Dosage form : —
Standard solution : Prepare solution of each drug substance in methanol.
Sample solution : Suitably dilute the sample with methanol for spotting.
Chromatographic conditions :

Test plate : Pre-coated TLC plate, silica gel SIL-G25

Format : 10 × 10 cm   *Thickness :* 250 µm

Volume spotted : 5 µl   *Separation technique :* Ascending

Mobile phase : Chloroform–acetone–methanol (55 + 35 + 10, v/v)

Chamber saturation : 15 min   *Migration distance :* 70 mm

Detection : Visible. Spray with 5% potassium dichromate solution in 10% sulphuric acid. After spray, allow the plate to dry in air—blue spots against greenish background are observed. 1% solution of potassium permanganate can also be used for detection.

HRf : Glycerin   20
         Ethylene glycol   35
         Propylene glycol   45
         Diethylene glycol   65

Comments : —
Reference : —

PROTOCOLS OF A THIN LAYER CHROMATOGRAM

Chromatogram No. 164

Formulation : Aflatoxin B_1, B_2, G_1, G_2

Classification : Miscellaneous

Dosage form : Almonds, peanuts, paprika

Standard solution : Dissolve the standard aflatoxin in acetonitrile for spotting.

Sample solution : Extract the powdered sample with methanol, filter and saturate with sodium chloride. Extract with petroleum ether. Reject ether layer and shake aqueous layer with dichloromethane. Evaporate dichloromethane layer and take up the residue in acetonitrile for application.

Chromatographic conditions :

Test plate : Pre-coated TLC plate, glass, SIL G-25-HR (M & N), or pre-coated HPTLC plate

Format : 10 × 10 cm   *Thickness :* 200 μm

Volume spotted : 1 μl   *Separation technique :* Ascending

Mobile phase :   1. Chloroform–acetone (90 + 10, v/v)
                   2. Chloroform–acetone–water (140 + 20 + 0.3, v/v)

Chamber saturation : —   *Migration distance :* 70 mm

Detection : Fluorescence 366 nm/> 400 nm

HRf :

	1	2
Aflatoxin B_1	75	47
Aflatoxin B_2	60	44
Aflatoxin G_1	55	42
Aflatoxin G_2	50	37

Comments : —

Reference : TLC Application Notes (M & N); Application Notes, p. 10, CBS-79, Sept. 97.

PROTOCOLS OF A THIN LAYER CHROMATOGRAM

Chromatogram No. 165

Formulation : Methanol, Ethanol, Propanol, Butanol, Amyl alcohol
Classification : Miscellaneous
Dosage form : —
Standard solution : —
Sample solution : —
Chromatographic conditions :

Test plate : Pre-coated TLC plate, cellulose-400 UV$_{254}$ (M & N)

Format : 5 × 10 cm   Thickness : 100 μm

Volume spotted : 5 μl   Separation technique : Ascending

Mobile phase : n-butanol–water–ammonia (50 + 40 + 10, v/v)

Chamber saturation : 10 min   Migration distance : 70 mm

Detection : UV (254 nm)—dark brown fluorescence

HRf :   Methanol   40
        Ethanol   50
        Propanol   65
        Butanol   75
        Amyl alcohol   85

Comments : —
Reference : TLC Application Notes (M & N), p. A-10.

PROTOCOLS OF A THIN LAYER CHROMATOGRAM

Chromatogram No. 166

Formulation : Thymol, Menthol, Eugenol, Carvacrol
Classification : Miscellaneous
Dosage form : —
Standard solution : —
Sample solution : —
Chromatographic conditions :

Test plate : Pre-coated TLC plate, silica gel 60W (Merck) or SiL-G25 (M & N)

Format : 5 × 10 cm   *Thickness :* 200 μm

Volume spotted : 1 μl   *Separation technique :* Ascending

Mobile phase : Toluene–chloroform (1 + 1, v/v)

Chamber saturation : 20 min   *Migration distance :* 60 mm

Detection : Visible. Spray with Emerson reagent, red spots against light yellow background or spray with anisaldehyde reagent.

HRf :   Thymol   30
         Menthol   15
         Eugenol   40
         Carvacrol   30

Comments : —
Reference : —

PROTOCOLS OF A THIN LAYER CHROMATOGRAM

Chromatogram No. 167

**Formulation : Propyl gallate, Octyl gallate, Butylhydroxyanisol (BHA), Butylhydroxy-
toluene (BHT)**

Classification : Miscellaneous (anti-oxidant)

Dosage form : —

Standard solution : —

Sample solution : —

Chromatographic conditions :

Test plate : Pre-coated TLC plate (glass), SIL G-25 (M & N)

Format : 5 × 10 cm   *Thickness :* 250 μm

Volume spotted : 2 μl   *Separation technique :* Ascending

Mobile phase : Petroleum ether (40-60)–toluene–glacial acetic acid (20 + 20 + 10, v/v)

Chamber saturation : 10 min   *Migration distance :* 70 mm

Detection : Visible. Spray with Gibb's reagent, heat at 105°C for 10 min and then expose
to ammonia vapours.

HRf :	Propyl gallate	10
	Octyl gallate	15
	BHA	60
	BHT	75

Comments : —

Reference : TLC Application Notes (M & N).

PROTOCOLS OF A THIN LAYER CHROMATOGRAM

Chromatogram No. 168

Formulation : Aspartame, Saccharin, Acesulfam

Classification : Miscellaneous (artificial sweeteners)

Dosage form : Syrup

Standard solution : Dissolve each substance in methanol for spotting.

Sample solution : For extraction of saccharin sodium, acidify the sample with 1 N sulphuric acid, extract with ether, evaporate ether layer and take up the residue in methanol for spotting.

Chromatographic conditions :

Test plate : Pre-coated TLC plate (glass), SIL G-25/UV$_{254}$

Format : 10 × 10 cm   *Thickness* : 250 µm

Volume spotted : 5 µl   *Separation technique* : Ascending

Mobile phase : 1. Acetone–toluene–glacial acetic acid (20 + 20 + 10, v/v)

2. Xylene–glacial acetic acid–n-propanol–formic acid (45 + 07 + 06 + 02, v/v)

Chamber saturation : 15 min   *Migration distance* : 70 mm

Detection : Spray with 0.2% ethanolic solution of dichlorofluoresceine sodium, followed by spraying with water and then view under UV (long).

HRf : Aspartame   10
        Saccharin   30
        Acesulfam   20

Comments : —

Reference : Application Notes (M & N), No. 167, p. A-77.

PROTOCOLS OF A THIN LAYER CHROMATOGRAM

Chromatogram No. 169

Formulation : Saccharin, Acesulfam, Cyclamate

Classification : Miscellaneous (artificial sweeteners)

Dosage form : —

Standard solution : —

Sample solution : —

Chromatographic conditions :

Test plate : Pre-coated HPTLC plate, cellulose (Merck)

Format : 10 × 10 cm   *Thickness :* 200 μm

Volume spotted : 5 μl   *Separation technique :* Ascending

Mobile phase : Ethyl acetate–acetone–ammonia (75 + 25 + 01, v/v)

Chamber saturation : 15 min   *Migration distance :* 2 × 70 mm (with
intermediate drying with warm air)

Detection : UV (365 nm) or spray with 0.1% solution of pinacryptol yellow reagent in
methanol.

HRf :   Saccharin   20 (violet colour)

      Acesulfam   30

      Cyclamate   10 (light orange)

Comments : —

Reference : —

PROTOCOLS OF A THIN LAYER CHROMATOGRAM

Chromatogram No. 170

Formulation : l-ornithine-l-aspartate

Classification : Miscellaneous

Dosage form : Tablets

Standard solution : Dissolve the peptide in formic acid for spotting.

Sample solution : Extract the powdered substance of the sample with formic acid for application.

Chromatographic conditions :

Test plate : Pre-coated TLC plate, silica gel 60F$_{254}$

Format : 10 × 10 cm　　　　　　*Thickness :* 250 μm

Volume spotted : 10 μl　　　　　*Separation technique :* Ascending

Mobile phase : n-butanol–water–glacial acetic acid (50 + 25 + 25, v/v)

Chamber saturation : 10 min　　　*Migration distance :* 70 mm

Detection : Visible. Spray with 0.5% ninhydrin solution in acetone, dry at 105°C for 10 min, look for two coloured spots corresponding to l-ornithine and l-aspartic acid.

HRf :　l-ornithine　　　　　　　23
　　　　l-aspartic acid　　　　　　36

Comments : —

Reference : —

PROTOCOLS OF A THIN LAYER CHROMATOGRAM

Chromatogram No. 171

Formulation : **Rutin Quercetin**

Classification : Miscellaneous

Dosage form : Tablets

Standard solution : —

Sample solution : —

Chromatographic conditions :

Test plate : Pre-coated TLC plate, silica gel $60F_{254}$

Format : 10 × 10 cm — *Thickness :* 250 µm

Volume spotted : 5 µl — *Separation technique :* Ascending

Mobile phase : Ethyl acetate–formic acid (98%)–water (85 + 10 + 15, v/v)

Chamber saturation : 30 min — *Migration distance :* 70 mm

Detection : Spray with 0.2% solution of aluminium chloride in methanol, air dry and dip in the solution of liquid paraffin + n-hexane (1 + 2) and examine fluorescent spot under UV (long)

HRf :		
	Rutin	30
	Quercetin	60

Comments : —

Reference : —

PROTOCOLS OF A THIN LAYER CHROMATOGRAM

Chromatogram No. 172

Formulation : Amaranth, Ponceau 4R, Erythrosine

Classification : Miscellaneous (food colours)

Dosage form : Syrups, tablets

Standard solution : Dissolve the different colours in dilute ammonia solution for application.

Sample solution : The sample is stirred with hot water until all the colour is extracted. Acidify with 1 M acetic acid, then add 3-4 de-greased undyed woollen threads. Boil for few minutes, remove the threads and extract the colours with dilute ammonia for spotting.

Chromatographic conditions :

Test plate : Pre-coated TLC plate, silica gel 60F$_{254}$

Format : 10 × 10 cm   *Thickness :* 250 μm

Volume spotted : 5 μl   *Separation technique :* Ascending

Mobile phase : Ethyl acetate–n-propanol–water (10 + 60 + 30, v/v)

Chamber saturation : —   *Migration distance :* 70 mm

Detection : Visible

HRf :   Amaranth (Pink)

          Ponceau 4R (Yellow)

          Erythrosine (Pink)

Comments : —

Reference : —

Glossary of TLC / HPTLC

Activity. Surface properties of a sorbent. The activity of a sorbent is affected by its water content which can be adjusted by relative humidity. Silica gel and aluminium oxide layers are activated at 105-110°C to desorb the physically bonded water. Aluminium oxide according to Brockmann is classified according to activity grades (I to V) depending on the residual moisture, grade V being the least active.

Adsorption chromatography. Chromatographic separation in a solid-liquid phase by competitive interaction between adsorption at the sorbent surface and dissolution in the moving mobile phase, resulting in separation of mixture according to the polarity of the individual components.

Anti-circular chromatography. Mobile phase moves from outside towards the centre of the circle. The samples are applied along the circle.

Chamber saturation. Before and during development, the components of the mobile phase are in equilibrium with the entire space in developing chamber. For uniform equilibrium, inside of the chamber is lined with filter paper on three sides. Usually Whatman filter No. 1 or of 3 mm thickness is used.

Chromatogram. Developed TLC plates (result of chromatographic separation), one may obtain photocopy, photograph or densitometric scan.

Chromatographic system. It comprises sample under analysis, sorbent (stationary phase) and eluent (mobile phase).

Circular chromatography. Mobile phase moves from centre towards outside, the samples are applied along a ring in the centre.

Clean-up. Process for removal of interfering matrix (excipients) from the sample for purification before subjecting to chromatographic analysis.

Densitometer. Chromatogram scanning spectrophotometer, usually called scanner, used for quantitative evaluation by recording absorbance or fluorescence in reflectance or transmission mode. The substance to be measured must either absorb light, stimulated to fluorescence or may be subject to post-chromatographic derivatization prior to evaluation.

Detection. Visualisation of separated substances after chromatographic development in order to assess their separation. Detection is based on specific colour of the substance, intrinsic fluorescence at 366 nm, property of fluorescence, quenching or post-chromatographic treatment of the plate with suitable colour reagent.

Development chamber. Glass trough chamber commercially available are commonly used for ascending chromatography. Chambers for horizontal or automatic development are available. Twin-trough chambers are suitable when equilibrating the layer is required.

Dyeing reagents. To detect colourless compounds which neither absorb in UV region nor have intrinsic fluorescent property. Dyeing reagents can be sprayed on the plate or the plate is dipped into them. 5% sulphuric acid in methanol, vanillin in sulphuric acid are the most common nonspecific dyeing reagents. One can use specific reagent such as ninhydrin for amino acid.

Edge effect. As TLC/HPTLC is an open system and if chamber is not adequately equilibrated, evaporation from edge of the plate causes Rf values of substances spotted on the outer sides of a plate to be higher than in the middle. This is called edge effect and can be prevented by equilibrating the chamber by lining with filter paper. One may avoid spotting of substances very close to the outer edges of the plates.

Eluent. Usually known as mobile phase.

Fluorescence. Molecules with rigid structures and π electron systems can be stimulated by radiation of suitable wavelength usually in UV region and emit radiation of lower energy, i.e., longer wavelength, mostly in visible region of the spectrum.

Fluorescence indicator. Such indicators are usually incorporated into the layers and make colourless substances visible by fluorescence quenching. Commonly used indicators are :

(i) F_{254} : Manganese-activated zinc silicate which when stimulated by short wavelength UV (254 nm) gives green fluorescence.

(ii) F_{254s} : Acid stable indicators usually useful in RPTLC when stimulated by short UV (254 nm) give pale blue fluorescence.

(iii) F_{366} : When stimulated by long UV (366 nm), intense blue fluorescence results. Optical brightners are commonly employed.

Fluorescence quenching. When the layers containing fluorescence indicators are stimulated by UV radiation (254 nm), colourless substances absorbing UV light appear as dark chromatographic zones on a green or pale blue fluorescent background-fluorescence indicator.

Forced flow technique. Movement of mobile phase under pressure or by centrifugal force in addition to the capillary forces present in the sorbent.

Gradient technique. Changing composition of the mobile phase during development (gradient elution or AMD technique).

HPTLC. High Performance Thin Layer Chromatography. In this case, the sorbent has finer particle size and the narrower distribution than conventional sorbents used for TLC. HPTLC layers are more homogeneous and thinner resulting in improved resolution, shorter analysis time, suitable for in situ quantitation.

Impregnation. Depending on the type of analysis layers are treated with liquid paraffin, buffers, acids, either by spraying or dipping for impregnation prior to development.

Horizontal development. Special development tanks which allow linear development from both sides of the TLC plates. This has advantage of high sample throughput.

Mobile phase. Solvent or mixture of solvents that move though the porous sorbent layers because of capillary action resulting in separation of substances under chromatographic analysis.

Multiple development. Development of chromatogram several times with intermediate drying of layer using the same mobile phase or different mobile phase. This brings about improvement in separation of complex mixtures such as that of amino acids (intermediate drying even at room temperature causes broadening of spots, resulting in diffusion).

Particle size. Smaller the particle size and narrower the distribution, better the separation efficiency. HPTLC plates have mean particle size of 4-6 µm whereas TLC plates have 10-12 µm.

Partition chromatography. Chromatographic development separation is based on solubility differences of individual components of a mixtures in mobile and stationary phases [layer of liquid (water) on the sorbent layer].

Preparative layer chromatograph (PLC). This technique is primarily used for purification and isolation of substances required for other chemical studies such as IR, GC, MS, NMR, etc. In this case, preparative plates with layer thickness of up to 2 mm are employed. The samples are applied as bands. The substance can be isolated by extracting the scrapped layer with suitable solvent.

Post-chromatographic. For detection of substances after development, the chromatogram is treated with suitable reagent, either by spraying or dipping. This is commonly known as post-chromatographic derivatization.

Pre-chromatographic. Subjecting substances to chemical derivatization prior to chromatographic separation.

Pre-coated layers/plates. When sorbent is coated as a thin layer on a suitable plate (glass, aluminium or plastic). The sorbent may contain suitable binder and fluorescent indicator. Layer thickness is usually 0.25 mm (TLC) 0.2 mm (HPTLC) or 0.5-2 mm (PLC).

Relative humidity. Degree of saturation of atmosphere with water at a particular temperature. It is possible to control the relative humidity with sulphuric acid solution of particular concentration or with saturated salt solution in contact with excess salt such as 25% sulphuric acid gives relative humidity of 65%, saturated solution of potassium chloride 85%, sodium chloride 75%.

Resolution. This is also called separation efficiency. This is judged by differences in Rf values of separated substances and conciseness of separated bands/spots. Band broadening, spot diffusion should be least for better resolution.

Retention factor (Rf). It is a parameter for qualitative analysis, i.e.,

$$Rf = \frac{\text{distance from starting line} \rightarrow \text{middle of spot}}{\text{distance from starting line} \rightarrow \text{solvent front}}$$

Rf values are between 0 - 1, best between 0.1 to 0.8 or 10-80 for HRf. Owing to the numerous effects influencing the migration of a substance, which are rather difficult to control all the times, Rf (HRf) should therefore be regarded as an approximate value. It is therefore desirable that a standard substance should be chromatographed on the same plate and under identical conditions. R_x or R_{st} value can be calculated as follows :

$$R_x \text{ or } R_{st} = \frac{\text{distance (starting zone – substance zone)}}{\text{distance (starting zone – zone of reference substance)}}$$

Rf value is always ≤ 1. R_{st} value can be > 1.0.

Reversed phases. Stationary phases (sorbent layers) are modified either by impregnating the normal layers with hydrophobic substances such as liquid paraffin or chemically modifying the layers by treatment with hydrocarbons such as alkyl chlorosilanes of different chain length. Common reversed phase plates (RP$_2$, RP$_8$, RP$_{18}$) are available. For such plates the mobile phases are predominantly polar-aqueous.

Sample application. After proper clean-up, the samples are applied to the starting line of a TLC plate. The samples may be applied either with the help of a syringe or capillary. However for quantitative TLC, the use of automated sample applicator is recommended for reproducible results.

Silica gel. Most commonly used sorbent; more than 80% chromatographic analyses are done using silica gel as stationary phase. It involves separation by adsorption and partition chromatography. Usually available in pore size of 40-60 Å (4 to 6 nm).

Sorbents. These can be inorganic such as SiO, Al$_2$O$_3$ or organic such as cellulose.

Surface area. Surface area of the sorbent expressed as m^2/g, includes both internal (surface area of pores) and external (surface area of particles), larger the surface area stronger will be the interaction between sample and stationary phase. Surface area in respect of silica gel 60 is 550 m^2/g whereas in case of silica gel 40 it is 750 m^2/g.

Stationary phase. Sorbent including any other molecule retained on its surface as a result of impregnation.

Stepwise development. Multiple development with mobile phase of graded polarity. Useful for separation of substances varying in their chromatographic behaviour (this is commonly referred as AMD technique).

Two-dimensional development. After first development, the chromatogram is dried and rotated through 90° and again subjected to ascending chromatographic development. One may use same or different mobile phases in two directions. This method is employed to improve separation of complex mixture or in validation of chromatographic conditions in respect of stability during spotting or development of a chromatogram.

Varo-KS chamber. These chambers are suitable for horizontal chromatography. For optimising the chromatographic conditions, several mobile phases alongside each other can be employed.

Literature

1. E.H. Deinstrop. J. Planar Chromatogr. *4*, 154-157, 1991.
2. E.H. Deinstrop. J. Planar Chromatogr. *5*, 57-61, 1992.
3. E.H. Deinstrop. J. Planar Chromatogr. *6*, 313-318, 1993.
4. K. Burger, J. Kohler and H. Jork. J. Planar Chromatogr. *3*, 504-510, 1990.
5. R.J. Maxwell, S.W. Yelsley and J. Unruh. J. Lig. Chromatogr. *13* (*10*), 2001-2011, 1990.
6. R.E. Kraiser. J. Planar Chromatogr. *1*, 182-187, 1988.
7. G. Windhorst and J.P. Delkleijin. J. Planar Chromatogr. *5*, 229-233, 1992.
8. N. Nurok. Chem. Rev. *89*, 363-375, 1989.
9. P.W. Paroch. J. Assoc. Off. Anal Chem. *53*, 530-534, 1976.
10. F. Abe and K. Sumejima. Anal. Biochem. *67*, 298-308, 1975.
11. K. Lee et al. J. Chromatogr. *174*, 187-195, 1979.
12. H. Bethke, W. Santi and R.W. Frei. J. Chromatogr. Sci. *12*, 392-97, 1974.
13. H. Jork, W. Funk W. Fischer and H. Wimmer. Thin layer chromatography, reagents and detection method. Vol. 1a & 1b. VCH Weinheim, FRG, 1990 and 1994.
14. K. Reuter, H. Knauf and E. Mutschlet. J. Chromatogr. *233*, 432-436, 1982.
15. Artz et al. J. Liq. Chromatogr. *3*, 1807, 1980.
16. Joseph Sherma, Whatman TLC Technical Services. Vol. 1, p. 20.
17. H. Halpaap, K.F. Krabs and H.E. Hauck J. High Resolution Chromatogr. *3* (*5*) 285-340, 1980.
18. R.E. Kaiser and R.J. Rider. J. Chromatogr. *142*, 411-420, 1977.
19. R.A. Elgi and S. Keller J. Chromatogr. 291, 249-256, 1984.
20. G. Szepesi. J. Planar Chromatogr. *6*, 187-197, 259-268, 1993.
21. K.F. Fodor, Z. Végh and Zs. Pap-Sziklay. J. Planar Chromatogr. *6*, 198-203, 1993.
22. Bernd Renger. Journal of AOAC, *76* (*1*), 7-13, 1993.
23. R.A. Elgi, H. Müller and S. Tanner. Anal. Chem. *305*, 267, 1981.
24. M. Prosek, M. Pukl, L. Miksa and A.G. Wondra. J. Planar Chromatogr. *6* (*1*), 62-65, 1993.
25. J. Sherma and B. Fried. Handbook of Thin Layer Chromatography Science, Series No. 55, Marcel Dekker, Inc., New York, 1991.
26. Bernard Fried and Joseph Sherma. Thin Layer Chromatography, Techniques and Application. 3rd ed. Marcel Dekker, Inc., 1994.
27. Bernard Fried and Joseph Sherma. Thin Layer Chromatography, Techniques and Application. Science Series, Vol. 66. Marcel Dekker, Inc., 1994.

28. P.E. Flinn, A.S. Kenyon and T.P. Layloff. J. Lip. Chromatogr. *15 (10)*, 1639-1653, 1992.

29. Ilkka Ojanpera et al. J. Lip Chromatogr. *14 (8)*, 1435-1446, 1991.

30. B. Pasciak. J. Planar Chromatogr. *5 (3)*, 205-206, 1992.

31. P. Duez, S. Chamart and M. Hanocq. J. Planar Chromatogr. *4 (1)*, 69-76, 1991.

32. Akira, Kunugi and Katsumi, T. Kagaku to Kyoiku, *42 (3)*, 206-210, 1994.

33. N. Nyiredy et al. J. Chromatography. *450*, 241-252, 1988.

34. Kang Jang Seong, Yakhak Hoechi, *38 (4)*, 366-71, 1994 (Korea).

35. G. Szepesi. Acta. Pharma. Hung. *61*, 67-76, 1991.

36. G. Szepesi, K. Gazdag and K. Mihályfi. J. Chromatogr. *464*, 265-278 and 279-289, 1989.

37. G. Szepesi, M. Gazdag, Zs. Pap-Sziklay and Z. Végh. J. Pharm. Biomed. Anal. *4*, 123-130, 1986.

38. J.C. Wahlich and G.P. Carr. J. Pharm. Biomed. Anal. *8*, 619-623, 1990.

39. P.A.D. Edwardson, G. Bhaskar, and J.E. Fairbrother. J. Pharm. Biomed. Anal. *8*, 929-933, 1990.

40. J.N. Miller. Analyst. *116*, 3-14, 1991.

41. E. Merck. HPLC/TLC/HPTLC Application Manual, 1986, Darmstadt, FRG.

42. Camag Bibliographic Service, Vol. 1-7, Muttenz, Switzerland.

43. H.E. Hauck, W. Jost, K.F. Krebs and F. Eisenbeiss. E. Merck (Chemical Reagents Division), Darmstadt, FRG.

44. W. Funk and P. Derr. J. Planar Chromatogr. *3*, 149-152, 1990.

45. Technical Aspects of HPTLC. Anchrom Enterprises (I) Pvt. Ltd., Bombay, Private Communication; 1994.

46. GLP in Chromatography. E. Merck, Technical Series, 1994.

47. Whatman Technical Series. Vol. 1, 2. 1981.

48. Whatman Technical Series. Vol. 3. 1982.

49. Whatman Chromatography Folios. Publication 842. TLCPS.

50. Merck Spectrum. 1994, pp. 1-36.

51. Thin Layer Chromatography, Application Manual. Macherey-Nagel (MN), Germany.

52. Thin Layer Chromatography; The Viable Alternative. TLC/HPTLC Application Notes. Macherey-Nagel (MN), Germany.

53. V.M. Shinde, B.S. Desai and N.M. Tendulkar. Indian Drugs, *31 (5)*, 192-195, 1994.

54. A.P. Argekar, S.V. Raj and S.U. Kapadia. Indian Drugs *32 (4)*, 166-171, 1995.

55. N.M. Tendulkar, B.S. Desai, V.M. Shinde. Abstract No. E8, 45th IPC, 1993.

56. M. El Sadek, A. El Shanawany, A. Aboul Khier and G. Rücker. Analyst, *115*, 1181-1184, 1990

57. V.M. Shinde, N.M. Tendulkar and B.S. Desai. J. Planar. Chromatogr. *7*, 50-52, 1994.

58. P.P. Shirke, M.K. Patel, V.M. Tamhane, V.B. Tirodkar. Indian Drugs *30 (12)*, 653-654, 1993.

59. P.P. Shirke, M.K. Patel, V.M. Tamhane, V.B. Tirodkar. Eastern Pharmacist, *37*, 155-156 and 179-180, 1994.

60. W. Funk, T. Kupper, A. Wirtz and S. Nitz. J. Planar. Chromatogr. *7*, 10-13, 1994.

61. P.P. Shirke, M.K. Patel, V.B. Tirodkar. Ind. J. Pharm. Sci., 108-109, 1994.

62. P. Parimoo, M. Mouniswamy, A. Bharathi, N. Lakshmi. Indian Drugs *31* (*5*), 211-214, 1994.

63. V.M. Shinde, N.M. Tendulkar, and B.S. Desai. J. Planar. Chromatogr., 7, 133-136, 1994.

64. Kajal Datta and S.K. Das. J. Planar. Chromatogr., 6, 204-207, 1993.

65. Joseph Sharma et al. J. Planar. Chromatogr., 3, 189-190, 1990.

66. V.M. Shinde, B.S. Desai, and N.M. Tendulkar. Indian Drugs, *31* (*3*), 119-121, 1994.

67. A.P. Argekar, S.U. Kapadia and S.V. Raj. Indian Drugs, *33* (*3*), 107-111, 1996.

68. A.P. Argekar, S.U. Kapadia and S.V. Raj. Indian Drugs, *33* (*3*), 167-170, 1996.

69. J.L. Chawla, R.A. Sodhi and R.T. Sane. Indian Drugs, *33* (*3*), 171-178, 1996.

70. J.L. Chawla, R.A. Sodhi and R.T. Sane. Indian Drugs, *33* (*5*), 208-212, 1996.

71. R.A. Sodhi, J.L. Chawla, and R.T. Sane. Indian Drugs, *33* (*6*), 280-285, 1996.

72. P. Parimoo, P. Priya, A. Bharathi and V.N. Mini. Indian Drugs, *33* (*7*), 329-333, 1996.

73. S. Chatterjee and B.P. Singh. Indian Drugs, *33* (*7*), 355-357, 1996.

74. R.A. Sodhi, J.L. Chawla and R.T. Sane. Indian Drugs, *33* (*12*), 601-603, 1996.

75. J.K. Lalla, S.U. Bhat, N.R. Sandu and M.U. Shah. Indian Drugs, *34* (*5*), 275-282, 1997.

76. J.L. Chawla, R.A. Sodhi and R.T. Sane. Indian Drugs, *34* (*6*), 339-345, 1997.

77. R.A. Sodhi, J.L. Chawla and R.T. Sane. Indian Drugs, *34* (*8*), 433-436, 1997.

78. S.S. Zarapkar, S.S. Kolte and S.H. Rane. Indian Drugs, *34* (*12*), 707-709, 1997.

Index